Food Saved Me

food
saved
me

My Journey of Finding
Health & Hope through
the Power of Food

danielle walker

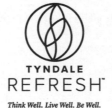

TYNDALE
REFRESH™

Think Well. Live Well. Be Well.

Visit Tyndale online at tyndale.com.

Tyndale and Tyndale's quill logo are registered trademarks of Tyndale House Ministries. *Tyndale Refresh* and the Tyndale Refresh logo are trademarks of Tyndale House Ministries. Tyndale Refresh is a nonfiction imprint of Tyndale House Publishers, Carol Stream, Illinois.

Food Saved Me: My Journey of Finding Health and Hope through the Power of Food

Designed by Libby Dykstra

Published in association with Yates & Yates (www.yates2.com).

Scripture quotations are taken from the *Holy Bible*, New Living Translation, copyright © 1996, 2004, 2015 by Tyndale House Foundation. Used by permission of Tyndale House Publishers, Carol Stream, Illinois 60188. All rights reserved.

The names and identifying details of the physicians and some of the other people who appear in this book have been changed to protect their privacy.

Source information for quotations, statistics, and resources is listed by page number in the endnotes section at the back of the book.

For information about special discounts for bulk purchases, please contact Tyndale House Publishers at csresponse@tyndale.com, or call 1-855-277-9400.

Library of Congress Cataloging-in-Publication Data

A catalog record for this book is available from the Library of Congress.

ISBN 978-1-4964-4474-5
ISBN 978-1-4964-6132-2 SPEC

Printed in the United States of America

27   26   25   24   23   22   21
7   6   5   4   3   2   1

For my grandma Marge.
You instilled an appreciation for family and community
in me from an early age; and you taught me what it looks
like to show affection through the food we make and the
conversations around our tables with the ones we love.

Contents

A Note from Me to You

This book is the story of how food saved my life. It's also a love story—about loving food, loving family, loving friends, and loving myself enough to take an active role in managing my own health. I have experienced a decade-long cycle of diagnosis, disease, remission, setbacks, recovery, and loss, but one thing has held true: Food continues to save me. And my mission is to help you understand all the different ways food can help save you, too.

If you have used my cookbooks or followed my blog or Instagram page for a while, you've probably read snippets of my story here and there, but until now, I've never done a deep dive. If you don't know me, let me introduce myself: I'm Danielle. I'm a wife, mom, and self-taught grain-free, gluten-free, and *mostly* dairy-free cook and baker from the San Francisco Bay Area.

When I was twenty-two, I was diagnosed with an extreme form of ulcerative colitis, an autoimmune disease that viciously attacks an otherwise healthy colon, resulting in severe—and in my case, life-threatening—malabsorption, malnutrition, and anemia.

In the first few years following my diagnosis, I was so sick I had to be hospitalized multiple times, and on more than one occasion, I required emergency blood transfusions and iron infusions just to stay alive. With each flare-up, my weight would fluctuate drastically. It wasn't unusual for me to lose as many as twenty to twenty-five pounds within a matter of weeks. That rapid weight loss would often lead to arthritis-like pain in all my joints, a ridiculously rapid heart rate, hair loss, energy loss, and a host of other problems.

Much to my dismay, my husband, Ryan, and I spent the better part of our first year as husband and wife in and out of emergency rooms and doctors' offices. We were unable to travel, stray too far from home, or even enjoy an evening out with friends and family for fear of what might happen if I had another flare-up.

In an attempt to manage my symptoms, my doctors prescribed high doses of steroids and other medications, the side effects of which were often as bad as, if not *worse* than, the disease itself. When I asked them whether food might affect my condition, each physician told me the same thing: "Diet didn't cause it, diet can't help it, and diet can't cure it." But as I continued relying solely on the prescriptions, my symptoms only worsened. My sickness controlled my life until I decided to take matters into my own hands and drastically change my diet.

After doing some research, I decided to stick to unrefined whole foods—the way people ate before the agricultural revolution changed the way food is grown and processed. I like to say it's the way humans were designed to eat before mass production ruined food and before convenience and immediate gratification largely displaced fresh, healthy, and real foods. My diet centers on grass-fed or pasture-raised proteins, fish, vegetables, fruit, seeds, nuts, and healthy fats. It eliminates dairy, legumes, grain products, sugar, gluten, and all processed food.

Almost immediately after I changed my diet, my symptoms began to subside, which was the sign of hope I needed to press forward. But virtually every dish I loved, growing up, had at least one if not multiple ingredients on my "can't have" list. That triggered a whole new list of fears and concerns:

Does this mean I'll never again be able to enjoy all the rich, creamy, sumptuous foods of my childhood?

Who's going to want to come to our house for a meal or a holiday celebration, knowing I'll only be serving grain-free, gluten-free, sugar-free, and dairy-free food?

Will people even feel comfortable inviting me to their homes and special events, knowing I probably can't eat what they're serving?

How will I eat when I'm traveling?

When I have children of my own, how will I pass down all of the food traditions and memories I grew up with?

My guess is that you have many of the same questions. And believe me, I get it. When you're forced to alter your diet drastically for the sake of your health, it's natural to worry that much of what makes life worth living will be lost along with your newly eliminated food groups. It's understandable to worry that you will miss out on special occasions with family and friends or be unable to provide homemade cookies for a child's party. And if you're anything like me, you're probably also worried that you'll never again be able to experience the joy that comes from lovingly preparing and serving food to the people you care about.

Well . . . over ten years, thousands of recipes, and three *New York Times* bestselling cookbooks later, I promise you, you *can* effectively manage your symptoms while still enjoying truly amazing food! The process may not be perfectly smooth, and you may hit bumps and setbacks like I have, but your entire life can change for the better.

When I embarked on this new food journey, I assumed it could only help those like me with digestive diseases. But since that day, I have received hundreds of thousands of emails and listened to personal accounts during my book tours from people all over the world who have experienced relief from everything from Crohn's disease, ulcerative colitis, multiple sclerosis, Hashimoto's disease, type 1 diabetes, rheumatoid arthritis, lupus, and psoriasis to autism, infertility, migraines, and food allergies. I've also received positive feedback from people without specific diagnoses whose brain fog, restless sleep, and everyday aches and pains cleared up after altering their diet. They're all managing their health while enjoying nutritious, great-tasting meals that even their friends and families love to eat.

Odds are, if you're reading this book, you or someone you know is struggling with some kind of autoimmune disease or other malady, and you're wondering if changing your diet can help. The short answer is yes! It most definitely can! The slightly longer answer lies in the pages that follow.

If you're new to grain-, gluten-, and dairy-free living, I want you to know that you're not alone. Hundreds of millions of people around the world suffer from various types of autoimmune diseases, and millions more from food allergies or chronic ailments. While diet may not provide a *complete* cure, changing how and what you eat *can* help you manage your health and significantly reduce both the frequency and the severity of flare-ups. I would bet my life on it. In fact, I have.

That's why I have written this book. I want to share my journey so that you will know that there is a path forward—there is healing and there *is* hope. In fact, if you take nothing else from my story, I pray it will be that—*there is hope*. Hope that you can live a full, happy, and healthy life without ever feeling hungry, excluded, or deprived. Hope that with each setback comes new learning and a renewed sense of determination. And hope that food *can* radically change your life for the better.

I know it can.

I've experienced it.

So have millions of others.

Now it's your turn.

Prologue

It was one in the afternoon, the Saturday before Thanksgiving 2009. In four hours, my husband, Ryan, and I were due at a friend's house for our annual "Friendsgiving," where we would celebrate the big day and feast with a few other newlyweds. After we were all sufficiently stuffed like turkeys, we would settle in for a competitive game of Dutch Blitz.

We always did it potluck style. The hostess would prepare the turkey and gravy, while everyone else was tasked with filling in the remaining Thanksgiving dishes—green bean casserole, cranberry sauce, stuffing, sweet potatoes with marshmallow topping, fluffy rolls with butter, crispy bacon-fried brussels sprouts, and of course, pumpkin and pecan pie.

This year, I had signed up for two items, but with trepidation. After spending two years suffering from a debilitating autoimmune disease that affected my digestion, I had vowed to completely overhaul the way I ate. It was an attempt to ditch at least some of the medications I was on, and with them, some of the symptoms I had been dealing with. I had just eliminated all breads, milk and butter, sugar, and some specific carbohydrates like white potatoes and other root vegetables that could be potential causes of inflammation.

Of course, when I made the decision, I hadn't thought about how difficult it would be trying to adhere to those new restrictions during an extremely food-focused holiday season. In retrospect, I probably should have put it off until the new year.

Most of my fondest memories were tied to holidays. And nearly all of them involved food. I so looked forward to gathering around the table with family and friends to enjoy one another's company over a wonderful meal. But now it all felt different. Lost. Abandoned. All those traditions felt like they were being discarded right alongside my newly rejected foods.

I sat in my kitchen looking at the dishes I had signed up to bring—mashed potatoes and a pumpkin pie—and realized I couldn't even eat them. I could make them "as is," so everyone *else* could enjoy them, but then what would *I* eat? Just the turkey and possibly a salad—without dressing or croutons—provided someone happened to bring one. That didn't sound at all like the joyful holidays I remembered so fondly.

Because mashed potatoes with loads of cream and butter is one of Ryan's favorite side dishes, I resolved to make them "as is" so he could pile his plate high with three scoops as usual, and make a second version for myself. I had read claims in low-carb, healthy recipe blogs and books that pureeing steamed cauliflower with some chicken stock was an even stand-in for mashed potatoes. It sounded a little far-fetched, but what other choice did I have?

So I printed out a recipe and went to work. I boiled the cauliflower and transferred the cooked florets to the mini food processor I'd received two years before as a wedding gift. It could hold only about a cup at a time, so I worked in batches, pulverizing the cooked florets into a white, creamy substance—a white, creamy substance that looked *nothing* like mashed potatoes with all their stature and texture. It was runny and lacked the billowy volume mashed potatoes have. It more closely resembled cauliflower soup.

I had followed the instructions to a T, so either that blog was fibbing, or the author hadn't eaten real mashed potatoes in years and had phenomenally low expectations. I, on the other hand, had just made the real deal and *accidentally* tasted a few bites as I was making them to check for flavor. And there was no tricking my taste buds.

The pie was a different story. There wasn't a stand-in for that. How could there be? Flour (gluten), butter and cream (dairy), and sugar. All things I couldn't eat. I made the pie from the recipe written in my grandmother's cursive on an index card, just as I had for years, and pushed past the disappointment that while everyone else was enjoying a slice of my past, I wouldn't be able to eat it. The autumnal smells of nutmeg and cinnamon wafting from the oven as the pumpkin custard baked were torturous, so I fled the room to shield my senses and set a timer upstairs so I wouldn't burn it. Actually, part of me kind of hoped it would burn, giving me a convenient excuse for not bringing it while avoiding the devastation of only being able to *smell* my favorite dessert of the season.

Shortly before four, Ryan loaded up our car with the creamy mashed potatoes, my cauliflower "soup," and the perfectly golden and set pumpkin pie before we made the ten-minute drive to our friends' home. When we arrived, the others were unloading their goodies, offering each other Thanksgiving hugs, and peeking under the foil at what others had brought.

"Don't worry. I brought real mashed potatoes too," I said as I registered the look on a few of my girlfriends' faces after they peered into my dish of cauliflower mush and took in the putrid smell that accompanies cooked cruciferous vegetables. I hadn't yet told our friends that I was embarking on this new way of eating, and I didn't want anyone to feel nervous about hosting us or guilty for eating my "off-limits" foods in front of me.

As a few of the ladies finished their remaining prep in the kitchen and set out some appetizers, the rest of the crew headed to the backyard for the annual game of touch football. As I sat watching the game, one of my friends set a basket of potato chips, a giant bowl of creamy onion dip, and a tray of cut vegetables surrounding a vat of ranch dressing on the bar next to me.

Potatoes are on my list of carbohydrates to cut out, I reminded myself, *so none for me.* The starches fed the bad bacteria in my gut, which I was trying to eliminate and replace with good, healthy bacteria that fight inflammation.

What is in that onion dip that I love so much? I thought as I eyed the carrots that I knew I *could* eat. I dreamt about smothering them in the creamy dip or drenching them in the ranch. *They probably have milk or sour cream in them—or both*, my brain reprimanded my growling stomach. *Dry carrots and celery it is.* I started munching on them like a bunny, eyeing with disdain the velvety dips that sat taunting me.

I heard the ding of the timer chime from the kitchen and walked inside to see our hostess pulling out the twenty-pound bird, roasted to golden perfection. She applied the final basting of juices and luscious fat that had dripped into the bottom of the pan, then tented the turkey and set it aside to rest while we guests displayed our reheated contributions on the countertop. Her husband did the honors and sliced the bird, presenting heaps of perfectly cooked dark and white meat on a platter adorned with citrus fruits and herbs.

Plates in hand, the gang ceremoniously lined up in the kitchen. I peered ahead of me, silently debating what I could and couldn't eat, and what *might* be okay just for tonight, even if it was technically off-limits. When I reached for a small spoonful of the golden, toasted stuffing wafting aromas of thyme and sage, Ryan gave me a gentle nudge. I'd told him on the car ride over not to let me slip up and eat the foods I had avoided over the last couple of months and vowed not to eat tonight, no matter how tempting.

While everybody else skipped my runny cauliflower soup, a poor stand-in for the buttery and creamy mashed potatoes that sat next to them, I ladled a few spoonfuls onto my plate. Like water flowing downhill, they cascaded out and filled my entire plate. As a kid, I hated when my foods touched on the plate. I had lightened up a bit as an adult, but I still preferred my sides and main dishes to have their own places. Apparently, the cauliflower "mashed potatoes" had a mind of their own.

I bypassed the green bean casserole, knowing that if it was anything like the one my sister and I were tasked to make growing up, it contained a can of cream of mushroom soup, a tub of sour cream, and onions coated in flour and fried until crisp. The canned soup likely included wheat and MSG, and it definitely included dairy. I swept over the sweet potatoes because they had golden browned sugar in them and toasted marshmallows on top; skipped the salad because it had croutons and more of that creamy ranch dressing; and didn't even look at the fluffy, warm dinner rolls and accompanying butter. It was just too cruel.

I finally got to the bird, picked out a few pieces of white meat— my favorite—and put them atop my cauliflower soup. The caramel-hewed pan gravy that sat in a boat next to the meat was calling my name, but I had seen the hostess whisking in cornstarch and wheat flour. I knew my body would not thank me later if I succumbed to its siren call. Having helped myself to all I could, I sat down at the table with my dry turkey and cauliflower soup and looked longingly at everybody else's plates heaped high with my seasonal favorites.

"How's it taste?" I asked Ryan.

"Horrible," he said with a half smile, knowing that's what I wanted to hear, even if it was the furthest thing from the truth.

While everyone else chattered away, raving about the food and complimenting each other on the different sides and dishes, I crawled into my own little hole. I felt different. Left out. Like everyone was looking at me. I felt sorry for myself. I didn't even have the courage to explain why I was eating this way for fear that we wouldn't be invited back to our friends' homes—or worse, that they wouldn't ever want to come to *our* house again.

I looked down at my plate of watery cauliflower. *In the US alone, millions of people suffer from autoimmune diseases and millions more have food allergies, and this is the best we can do? This terrible food that sucks the joy out of us?* I couldn't stand the thought that this was what I would be reduced to eating if I wanted to be healthy.

Why not create your own recipes then? I mused.

I *did* like to cook, but I mostly made simple dishes, and I worked from recipes my mom and grandmas had been using for years. I had never created my own recipes before.

Still . . . , I thought, lifting my fork and watching the diluted soup drip back down onto my plate, *whatever I come up with couldn't be any worse than this.*

PART 1

Love Well

1

I have *always* loved food.

Many of my favorite childhood memories center around meals or treats. Whose don't? For me, the best memories are of my parents, siblings, and me eating big family dinners and celebrating every holiday imaginable at my grandparents' house.

From as far back as I can remember, twenty to thirty of us would gather at my grandparents' house for a feast every month. My sweet Italian grandmother, Grandma Marge, made everybody feel loved and cared for through food. She always had an extensive buffet of homemade *everything*—at least three different meats, roasted salmon, freshly made tortellini with homemade marinara, a huge salad, steamed artichokes and asparagus, rolls, pies, fudge-swirled vanilla ice cream, and her famous fruit crisps.

I especially remember the big family crab feeds she hosted each winter. Dungeness crab, which is in season then, is big in the San

Francisco Bay Area where I am from. When my cousins, siblings, and I were really little, Grandma Marge would crack the crab for all eight of us and have it waiting on our plates while the adults labored over their dinners. She definitely knew how to spoil us!

When I got older and was able to crack open the shells myself, I followed the way my family did it. Everybody was quiet while we concentrated on releasing the succulent meat from the reddish-orange shells. All you could hear was *crack, crack, crack*. We cracked for what seemed like an eternity without so much as a taste so we could feast on that huge stack of crab meat all at once. And my family *loves* mayonnaise, so bowls of mayo would be scattered around everywhere for us to dip the meat in. It was heavenly!

It wasn't just the food that made everything so special; it was celebrating and connecting with family and friends. Enjoying good food with loving people made me feel like I belonged. And at the center of all of it was Grandma Marge, the delighted hostess making sure that everyone felt important, needed, and loved.

What impressed me most, though, wasn't how sweet Grandma Marge was or how delicious her food was, but how simple she made it all look. And believe me, it wasn't. She never allowed potlucks at her house. She made every single dish fresh and from scratch. Nothing from a box! And she accepted help from no one. It didn't matter if someone was a vegetarian, a pescatarian, or was allergic to dairy, she had something for each of us—her special ingredient... love—and I wanted to be just like her someday.

When I was five, my family moved away from the Bay Area to Colorado. We continued to go to Grandma Marge's whenever we were in town, but I missed those monthly feasts with our extended family so much. Because we didn't have family in Colorado, my parents focused on growing our circle of friends through church and my dad's work, and my mom took over the hosting duties, which she loved. We called these new friends our extended family and spent most of our holidays and special occasions with them.

Mom worked outside of the home, so she didn't have time to cook everything from scratch. But her meals were still delicious, especially the velvety casseroles enriched with a couple of cans of cream of mushroom soup, a tub of sour cream, and a layer of cheese on top, as well as the French dip sandwiches with thinly sliced roast beef piled high on crusty rolls, blanketed in gooey cheese and mayo, with a bowl of brackish dipping juice on the side.

When my sister, Leisa, and I were old enough to help in the kitchen, those were the first treasured recipes she taught us to make. She also taught me some recipes from her mom, Grandma Bonnie. I still relish the taste of Grandma Bonnie's very Americanized version of a shepherd's pie, which we made frequently—ground beef layered with thin French green beans and a box of dried flaked mashed potatoes, all smothered in a creamy sauce of cream of mushroom soup and sour cream, and covered in cheese and fried onion strings.

Sundays were for tacos. As soon as the church service ended, my sister and I changed out of our Sunday dresses and headed into the kitchen to help Mom with the preparation. I mastered the art of browning the ground beef and stirring in a packet of seasoning by the time I was ten, and we all helped with chopping and prepping the fixings—lettuce, tomatoes, refried beans, grated cheese, sour cream, and black olives. We'd lay all of the bowls heaped with toppings out on a lazy Susan set in the middle of the table. Most Sundays we shared the meal with our "extended family."

Where Mom really outdid herself, though, was in celebrating holidays. She learned that from her mom, and she left no stone unturned. Every Valentine's Day, our breakfast table was blanketed with a big box of See's chocolate hearts, pink pancakes, and toad-in-the-hole (an egg fried in the heart-shaped hole cut from a piece of bread). My sister, brother, and I would squeal with delight when we entered the kitchen for breakfast on St. Patrick's Day and spotted a box of Lucky Charms with green shamrocks adorning the table. And on Halloween, Count Chocula cereal and powdered-sugar doughnuts started our day on a festive note. That evening, before we would put on our costumes and head out to nab a ton of sugary treats, Mom would cook up pumpkin soup and hamburgers—a mash-up of traditions from Grandma Bonnie and Grandma Marge.

Christmastime was my favorite. The day after Thanksgiving, we decorated every inch of our house, and all month long we watched every sappy Christmas movie we could find on television while baking dozens upon dozens of cookies to give away as presents—cutout sugar cookie reindeer, bells, Santas, and stars, all covered with red-and-green icing and sprinkles; spicy gingerbread men with little red cinnamon eyes and buttons; rich chocolate fudge squares made with a jar of marshmallow fluff; thumbprint shortbread cookies filled with different flavors of sweet jam; gingersnaps; biscotti; and creamy peanut butter balls dipped in dark velvety chocolate.

The cornerstone of Christmas breakfast was Grandma Marge's braided cinnamon swirl loaf. She would spend the entire week mixing, kneading, proofing, and baking enough loaves to give one to each of her kids and their families, always making a handful of extras to distribute to extended family and friends. In between the crusty pieces of braided dough hid a hot, sticky center laced with a hefty dose of cinnamon. And when she pulled it out of the oven, she drizzled it with a snow-white powdered sugar glaze. She had to have made at least two dozen individual loaves each year. Even after we moved, she continued to ship them to us.

Come Christmas Day, my dad would take over, using recipes he had learned from Grandma Marge and *his* grandmothers—Granny Sarella and Grandma Ruby. Though I don't remember seeing him cook much during my childhood, I do vividly remember the meal he made every Christmas—standing rib roast with caramelized onions, roasted sweet carrots, and potato wedges; a pan gravy made with a roux and lots of pepper and garlic; salad with bay shrimp doused in his favorite blue cheese dressing; and butter-and-garlic-drenched mushrooms and zucchini. He cooked all day while my siblings, Leisa and Joel, and I played with our new toys.

As we grew older, we started to find our way around the kitchen a bit better ourselves and took full advantage of our small bit of knowledge to make some extra cash. We were always creating *something* to sell—from beaded necklaces, friendship bracelets, and homemade pillows to our very creative lemonade concoction called "Fizzy Coolers" (made with a proprietary mix of lemonade, Sprite, and Kool-Aid). Our entrepreneurial brains were constantly looking for ways to earn an extra dollar or two. Our favorite was when we played restaurant and offered a date night of sorts to our parents. For a hefty dollar, we sold them a simple dinner of food they had purchased and we had put together. We would don our parents' oversized adult aprons, light a candle on the table, throw on some Frank Sinatra, and sketch out the menu on the meal-plan chalkboard Mom had hanging in the kitchen. I would usually play maître d', while Leisa played the server and Joel was the food runner.

When I was fifteen, Dad got a new job and we returned to the Bay Area. While I was thrilled at the prospect of being able to take part in Grandma Marge's regular feasts once again, Colorado had become my home. I was about to enter my sophomore year of high school, had campaigned for and been elected to student council, and had made the varsity lacrosse team. I finally felt like I had a group of friends I could trust and with whom I looked forward to spending my final three years of high school. Now that was all being ripped away.

The angst I felt—and subjected my poor parents to—lingered throughout my sophomore year. Then one evening the summer before my junior year, a friend brought a group of us together with a bunch of her guy friends from a rival high school the next town over. One in particular caught my eye.

"Who's that?" I asked, eyeing the cute, brown-haired guy with bleached blond tips and bright blue eyes leaning up against a raised red Jeep Cherokee covered in snowboarding bumper stickers.

"That's Ryan Walker," my friend whispered back.

"Oh my gosh, he's so hot!" I couldn't remember the last time I blinked.

"You don't know the half of it," she continued. "He's captain of the football team, and rumor has it, he's a shoo-in for homecoming king."

Ryan Walker. "Oh, that's the guy Christa went on a date with," I said. I felt a little deflated as I realized that he might already be taken.

I must have made some kind of impression on Ryan that first night because a few weeks later, when he went off to snowboarding camp, he called me every night. (Apparently things were over with the other girl.) We got to know each other over the phone, and with every call, I liked him more and more. While funny and outgoing, he seemed to have a good head on his shoulders and focused on football and school over partying.

And even though Ryan was an only child, his family sounded a lot like mine. His parents went to every one of his football games, just like mine went to all my lacrosse games, and they were as big into hospitality as my parents were, always welcoming his friends into their home.

When he got home from camp, he asked me out. I was thrilled to say the least. And as an added bonus, while he was gone, I'd gotten my braces removed! We went on a few dates that summer, but ultimately broke up so he could enjoy his senior year—and date the cheerleader at his school that everyone said he should. Oh, high school! But we stayed close, and our friendship blossomed.

I pursued him like a moth to a flame his entire senior year. I even went to *two* different proms my junior year with two of his good friends, hoping it would make him jealous (earning me the affectionate nickname "Walker Stalker" from my friends)!

Then, just when I had all but given up hope that Ryan felt the same way I did, a group of us went to Yosemite right after his graduation. We loaded into that red raised Jeep and made the four-hour drive to the beautiful valley floor where we had reserved a camping spot. We all pitched in making dinner around the campfire. We cooked hot dogs on skewers, heated baked beans on a little propane burner, and because my mom always made tuna casserole when we camped, I treated everyone to the timeless delicacy that is egg noodles, a tin of Chicken of the Sea, and a can of cream of mushroom soup. After dinner, Ryan and I hiked to the top of a big boulder to look at the clear sky, which was studded with tiny golden stars. We started talking about his upcoming freshman year at the University of Colorado. Because I had grown up in the state, he loved asking me all about it.

That's when it happened.

"I'm falling in love with you," he said.

"You are?" I said in disbelief. No one had ever said those words to me before. "I feel the same. I've been falling in love with you for the past year."

We spent the rest of the evening lying on that big boulder, talking about his imminent departure for another Boulder, and how we could possibly work things out with the distance. We drove home a couple of days later and spent the rest of that summer attached at the hip. I worked at a P.F. Chang's that was right down the street from his parents' house. I would head there after work and eat the leftover dinner his mom always saved for me. I loved Ryan's parents, and God bless them, they treated me like the daughter they never had.

That fall, Ryan headed off to Colorado for college, and we both wept as we said goodbye and ended our relationship. It's not that we wanted to; we just assumed that's what you did when one of you was starting college and the other one was stuck in her final year of high school. Ryan wrote me love letters via e-mail daily during his first few weeks away. I, in turn, was miserable without him and didn't want to be part of anything fun or exciting at school. After about a month of silently pining for one another, we cracked, tearfully confessing to each other that we couldn't bear the thought of either of us being with anyone else, and embarked on a year of long-distance dating.

The following fall, I enrolled at Colorado State University in Fort Collins, executing the plan I'd had in my head since first moving back to California—to attend the same college where my sister was completing her final year. I was now about an hour north of Ryan.

One weekend early in my freshman year, I decided to do something a little special for Ryan and his roommates.

"I'm going to make chicken Parmesan for you guys this weekend," I announced. Granted, I had never made it before, but I'd seen people make it on television, and it was one of my favorite things to order when I went out to eat at Buca di Beppo. To be honest, I don't even think I had a recipe. I just figured, *How hard can it be? It's just spaghetti and breaded chicken.*

The guys were thrilled. After all, it's not often you get a real home-cooked meal when you're away at school. They even chipped in to help buy the ingredients.

As soon as I arrived at their apartment, I shooed them all out of the kitchen and got to work. I coated the thick boneless chicken breasts in an egg wash and Italian bread crumbs mixed with grated Parmesan and fried them in a pan on the stove, just like I'd seen on TV. After turning each one a couple of times, I noticed the breading was starting to burn, so I pulled them off the heat and stuck the pan in the oven to keep everything warm while I made the pasta. Once the pasta was ready, I pulled the pan out, placed the chicken breasts atop the pasta, and added a few slices of mozzarella and a sprinkle of Parmesan cheese. I placed the pan under the broiler just long enough for the chicken to become bubbly. Then I heated up a jar of marinara sauce to blanket the cheesy chicken and proudly served it to the boys.

It looked and smelled amazing.

The boys eagerly grabbed their knives and forks and immediately started digging into the chicken. Then, one by one . . . they stopped.

What's the matter? I asked.

After exchanging a few awkward glances, Ryan finally spoke up. "Um, this isn't cooked."

"What?" I grabbed his plate and inspected the beautifully golden chicken. Sure enough, the inside wasn't just pink; it was 100 percent raw. I had no idea that after you seared the chicken to get a good crust, you had to *cook* it the rest of the way in the oven—*or* that you were supposed to pound the chicken flat before you breaded it so it would cook evenly.

I was mortified. After apologizing profusely, I collected all of their plates and cooked the chicken the rest of the way through.

That first failure sparked a hunger within me to get it right. I began religiously reading cooking magazines, watching the Food Network, and imitating the likes of Rachael Ray, Ina Garten, and Giada De Laurentiis. I might not have had their pedigree, skill level, or equipment, but after nearly poisoning the love of my life, I was determined that at the very least, the next time I cooked for someone, the food would not be raw.

Despite the fact that I almost killed him, Ryan still saw a future for us, and we talked about marriage almost daily. He even burned me a CD and attached a little sticker of a bride and groom to the top where he wrote "you" and "me" with arrows pointing to the happy couple. Next to that was a handwritten note and the sequence of songs he'd included.

But while we were both desperate to move forward with our relationship, share a home, and never have to say goodbye at night, Ryan's parents felt otherwise. They were 100 percent *for* us. They just didn't want us to make the mistake of marrying too young, so they said that if we got married before we graduated, they would stop paying Ryan's tuition. Neither of us wanted to see that happen. We were young, but we were smart enough to know that going into a marriage with two college tuition loans to pay off could cause some newlywed turmoil. I knew Ryan had looked at rings and had been saving up what little money he had. And we *talked* about getting engaged constantly. Still . . . I hated waiting.

Because we knew that eventually we wanted to settle in California (not being fans of Colorado's harsh winters), we transferred to different colleges in Southern California to finish our degrees the semester after the raw chicken fiasco.

During my junior year of college, in December of 2005, Ryan and I planned to head to Maui with his parents right around Christmastime. He knew what a fanatic I was about Christmas, and given the romantic setting, I had an inkling he might propose.

Each day he gave me a note or memento from our relationship centered around the theme of "The Twelve Days of Christmas"— apartment listings from Southern California, a ticket from a USC football game, a gas receipt from our numerous drives up I-5 to visit our families in Northern California on holidays. Because we were only going to be in Maui for eight days, I assumed that if he was going to propose, it would be on day seven. So on day six, I painted my nails with a fresh coat of polish—you know, just in case I was about to get a new ring to show off. That day, Ryan sent me to the hotel spa for my first ever professional massage and facial. It was dreamy.

We had dinner plans that evening, but when I got back from the spa, Ryan told me his parents needed more time to get ready and suggested we go for a walk on the beach. It was beautiful. The sun was about to set as we walked barefoot, hand in hand, down the Kaanapali beachfront. About twenty minutes in, we turned around to head back. Suddenly Ryan stopped and took both my hands in his. *What's happening?* My mind raced. *This isn't supposed to happen until day seven!*

The next thing I knew, Ryan got down on one knee and pulled out a little box with Ashley Morgan written on it. I knew that name. She was a friend of my sister's. She was also a jewelry designer and had made Leisa's custom engagement ring.

"Danielle," he said, his eyes misting over, "I love you more than life itself, and I cannot imagine spending my life without you. I know you have been waiting for this, maybe even *expecting* it tomorrow, so I had to throw you off and do it today." He laughed, then held my hand tighter. "Danielle Lynne Norsworthy, will you marry me?"

Tears flooded my eyes, and my already sunburned cheeks turned an even brighter shade of red.

"Yes!!! A million times, yes!" I screamed in excitement.

He rose from his knee and picked me up, twirling me around in the setting sun while the waves came crashing in behind us.

Then he carried me over to the grass, where his parents were waiting with a bouquet of flowers and a camera.

That night at dinner, I couldn't stop looking at the gorgeous ring he'd designed. A Royal Asscher cut—my favorite because it had a vintage appeal and beautiful square shape with rounded edges and layered facets. When you look deep into the diamond from the top, it's like looking into a kaleidoscope. It was set in a platinum band, and on the interior, he'd had our initials engraved. Everything about it was perfect.

By the way . . . day seven's gift? Getting to spend the rest of my life with my best friend.

2

"You seem pretty excited," Ryan said, smiling as he pulled his freshly washed car into the clubhouse parking lot on a sunny Saturday in late July.

"I am!" I smiled back. What *wasn't* there to be excited about? In just over a month, I would be marrying the love of my life, and I was about to spend a picture-perfect afternoon celebrating with family and friends at a bridal shower hosted by Grandma Marge.

The last few months had been a whirlwind of activity. Ryan had passed his LSATs and was getting ready to start law school. I'd just completed my last semester of college—studying for finals and completing an internship with a public relations firm while working part-time as a server at a local restaurant. I was also trying to find a place for us to live *and* plan a wedding! As much as I was enjoying watching the details of our future fall into place, I had to admit that the stress and lack of sleep were starting to take their toll. Plus, earlier that summer, I'd gotten hit with a horrific stomach bug that I couldn't seem to shake, despite a full round of antibiotics. But I was determined to set all the anxiety and uncertainty of the past three months aside. Today was all about sitting back, enjoying time with family and friends, and—knowing Grandma Marge—partaking in a spectacular spread.

"Okay, here we are," Ryan said, stopping in front of the clubhouse entrance. "You have fun today, okay?" He leaned in and gave me a quick kiss.

"You too!" I said, giving his hand a final squeeze before jumping out of the car.

While I was off celebrating with the girls, Ryan would be taking in a round of golf with my dad; my brother, Joel; and Leisa's husband, Tyson. He'd been looking forward to it for weeks, and I just loved seeing how beautifully our families got along. Yep, everything was turning out perfectly.

As soon as I walked into the clubhouse, I was met by an excited chorus of squeals and bear hugs from grandmas, aunts, cousins, future in-laws, and girlfriends. My mom has always been very social, the life of the party, so *everybody* is her best friend. As a result, most of my friends were the daughters of *her* friends, and virtually all of them were there.

Grandma Marge had decked out the entire dining area in red and white. There were red and white carnations in cute little bud vases in the center of every table; pristine, starched white tablecloths on every table; and white crepe paper wedding bells hanging from all the chandeliers. It wasn't *quite* the USC Trojan burgundy I had selected for our wedding color in honor of Ryan's alma mater, but it was beautiful.

I was especially drawn to the photos of Ryan and me, which adorned the walls like a giant scrapbook of our relationship. There were baby photos, pictures of us as little kids, shots of us hiking and skiing together in Colorado, prints of the two of us cuddling in the stands at USC football games, spending holidays with our families, our trips to Yosemite and Maui, and our engagement photos—five years' worth of memories, and a lifetime yet to go.

We all mingled for a bit, munching on chips and Grandma's signature garlic–cottage cheese dip while we caught up with what everyone had been doing since graduation that spring. Then after Grandma Marge peeled back the sheets of aluminum foil from the platters lining the buffet table, we ate.

As anticipated, Grandma Marge had pulled out all the stops. Everything was homemade, and she included all my favorites—her famous curry chicken salad served atop an enormous bed of lettuce; shrimp cocktail; marinated artichoke hearts; penne pasta with her homemade marinara; braised chicken with mushrooms; and a colossal watermelon, hollowed out like a bowl and filled with sliced fruit and fresh berries. Rounding out those dishes was a plate of Hawaiian sweet rolls, my grandma Bonnie's signature red Jell-O salad with fruit and marshmallows, and a white Pyrex dish brimming with Italian marinated three-bean salad from Costco— a family favorite.

After everyone enjoyed the feast, we gathered around the pile of brightly wrapped presents stacked in front of the fireplace. To make things interesting, my sister arranged a round of wedding gift bingo, where everyone fills in their squares with gifts they think the bride will get and marks them off as they go. Those who knew me well—which was pretty much everyone in the room—wisely filled their cards with kitchen sets, cookware, and baking accessories. They *knew* how eager I was to outfit my first kitchen with the same shiny pots, pans, and utensils I was forever *oohing* and *aahing* over while watching the Food Network. The fact that I also worked part-time at Pottery Barn throughout college (and next door to their sister company, Williams-Sonoma) and had been regaling them with descriptions of all my favorite kitchen gizmos and gadgets for months didn't hurt their chances either.

Not that I'd actually *done* much cooking, mind you. Aside from a handful of basic recipes I'd learned from my mom, the extent of my cooking prowess was basically crushing up frozen hamburger patties, browning them in a pan, and then stirring the meat into a bowl of boiled spaghetti noodles and dousing it with a jar of store-bought marinara sauce. To be fair, I made a mean garlic bread to go with it, which pretty much amounted to cutting a French loaf in half (why I didn't at least use Italian bread, I have no idea), spreading butter on it, and then sprinkling it with garlic salt. That's what my mom made on spaghetti night as I was growing up, and Ryan loved when I made it. I'd always figured I would venture into cooking and baking more once I got married, since I was hoping to eventually be able to cook—and host—like Grandma Marge. The first step? A fully stocked kitchen. And, of course, recipes.

Because so many of our family traditions centered around food, Mom and Grandma Marge had asked everyone to include a favorite family recipe with their gift. Some people tied the recipe to the gift thematically, which gave me a better understanding of how to use the tool. My mom, for instance, wrote out the shepherd's pie recipe she'd taught me as a little girl and gave it to me along with a Pyrex casserole dish. She also gave me ramekins to hold the au jus in her recipe for French dips. Even though I'd made both dishes enough times to memorize the recipes, there was something about seeing them written out in my mom's handwriting that made them extra special.

Ryan's mom gave me a gorgeous cherry-red Le Creuset Dutch oven with a ceramic exterior and cast-iron interior, along with her own mother's beef stew recipe.

"You're marrying my son," she said as I quickly perused the recipe before handing it over to my sister, who was arranging them all in a three-ring binder. "This is his favorite meal." Unfortunately, I never got to meet Ryan's grandma. She passed away before we started dating. So to be able to make him his favorite meal of hers . . .

"Thank you so much," I said. "Ryan will absolutely love this! He always tells me about Nanny's beef stew and her famous butter-filled mashed potatoes."

"Just remember," she cautioned me, "you practically have to burn the beef. If it's not blackened and sticking to the bottom of the pan, you're not browning it long enough."

I was fairly confident I could burn stew meat. And I'd eaten enough beef stew to know that the sauce did, in fact, taste much richer and fuller when it contained all the delicious little baked-on bits that you scrape off the bottom of the pan with a wooden spoon and add to the beef broth.

Next up was my grandma Bonnie's famous German sour meatball recipe, which came to me nestled in the bottom of a stainless-steel stockpot. I know. *Sour* meatballs don't sound very appetizing, but these were amazing, and they were even better when you stopped to consider the love that went into making them.

Grandma Bonnie's hands were completely gnarled due to her rheumatoid arthritis, yet every time we had a family get-together, she would hand-crush an entire sleeve of saltines, mix them in with ground beef and eggs, and then compress them into perfect little golf ball–sized meatballs, which she would simmer for an hour in water with a few bay leaves and whole allspice. The sour part of the dish—her yellow-mustard gravy—would come together with a roux of butter and flour, a few ladles of beef broth from the meatballs, mustard, and apple cider vinegar. The meatballs would be added to the gravy and rolled around until they were fully coated, then served over a heap of mashed potatoes with an extra spoonful of the sour gravy. Making them had to be excruciating for her, but the end result was the stuff of legend. My brother, Joel, and I used to compete to see how many we could eat. His max was fifteen (I'm proud to report I never even came close).

The crowning glory of our family's recipes, though, had to be my grandma Marge's famous tomato meat sauce. Just the slightest step up from my crumbled-up frozen hamburger patties and a jar of sauce from Trader Joe's, which took less than fifteen minutes to throw together, Grandma's meat sauce simmered for four full hours on the stove. At the bottom of the pot was a bone-in pork chop, which when simmered long and slow, released a subtle pork flavor and allowed the collagen and gelatin in the bones to enrich and thicken the sauce. She would remove it at the very end, just before sprinkling in her mom's secret ingredient—a pinch of cinnamon. As the story goes, whenever her mother, Granny Sarella, would make this sauce, the men in the family would fight over who got to eat the pork chop when it came out of the pot, and I don't blame them. When that chop came out, the meat would literally be falling off the bone and dripping in sauce.

When we moved to Colorado, my mom made her own version of Grandma Marge's meat sauce, adding diced green bell peppers, button mushrooms, and a couple of glugs of red wine. Instead of simmering it on the stove all afternoon, she made it in the Crock-Pot. It was excellent, but believe me, she took a lot of flak over those modifications from our extended family.

"That's not the real recipe," they would tell her. "We drink the wine while we make it; we don't put it in the sauce!"

Well . . . now *I* had the real recipe. And in Grandma Marge's own handwriting. How she managed to get it down, I'll never know, since she never actually measured anything. It was all in her head—a pinch here, a dash there, a handful, a splash, a glug—it must have taken my mother hours to settle on the right amounts with her, which made the gift all the more special.

After the gifts were opened, we tucked into dessert—thirty-five little lemon cakes covered in velvety white icing with tiny edible flower decorations, each topped off with two scoops of lemon ice cream. And because she knew how much I preferred chocolate over lemon, Grandma had also made a full-size heart-shaped chocolate Bundt cake, dusted with powdered sugar and adorned with a vintage bride-and-groom cake topper from her own wedding back in 1956.

It was a perfect day, filled with love and laughter, but by the time Ryan picked me up, I was completely exhausted.

"You still not feeling 100 percent?" he asked, a tinge of concern in his voice as we pulled out onto the freeway, gifts piled high in the back seat.

"I'm sure it's just from all the running around getting ready for the wedding. And I definitely overate today," I said, stifling a laugh. "It'll pass." I leaned over and kissed his cheek. "Everything's going to be just fine."

And it was. We were married on September 2, 2007, in the charming Presidio Chapel, located on a picturesque former army base in San Francisco. The wedding was every bit as beautiful as I had imagined, and when the officiant—who happened to be my dad—said, "I now pronounce you husband and wife," I literally jumped up and down for joy. I'm sure every bride feels this way, but everything about our ceremony and reception at the gorgeous Golden Gate Club was perfect—from the rigorously tested and designed menu to the signature pomegranate crimson cocktail we created to match our wedding colors—everything went smoothly. After five years of dating, a two-year engagement, a few different colleges, and a handful of moves, we were finally Mr. and Mrs. Ryan Walker. I'd never felt so alive and loved.

Thankfully, before the wedding someone advised us to have the caterer set aside some appetizers for the wedding party since they usually miss out on the cocktail hour due to photos. Best advice ever—my stomach was feeling a little off from all the nerves and excitement, but more than anything, I was famished! So once the photography session wrapped up and our guests took to the dance floor, which was adorned with a lit-up monogram of our name and featured a picturesque view of the Golden Gate Bridge out the floor-to-ceiling windows, Ryan and I munched on flank steak–wrapped asparagus, chicken sliders, and stuffed mushrooms. After that, we were right with our guests on the dance floor enjoying the band and our favorite thing—dancing. Ryan is like the Energizer bunny on the dance floor. He long outlasts me, and my mom's friends were asking my permission to have a spin with him on the floor while I took a break and showed off my ring to guests.

After we said our final goodbyes and changed into our getaway outfits, Ryan and I jumped into his mom's convertible and headed out for our honeymoon, which was actually more of a mini-honeymoon. Ryan had already started his law classes at the University of California Hastings, so instead of having a full-blown honeymoon right away, we simply drove north across the Golden Gate and forty minutes into wine country to spend a few days in the Napa Valley, with plans to enjoy private tastings and vineyard tours. Even though it was short, our mini-moon was everything we intended it to be, and we enjoyed the best food and wine Napa Valley could provide.

Afterward, we settled into our new apartment to begin life together. We'd found a charming little duplex in Lafayette, a suburb of San Francisco, and I quickly set about making it a home, dreaming of the day when we could begin hosting our own family get-togethers. We had a small brick courtyard out back, and I couldn't wait to start working on the grassy area behind it, where I would grow my very own tomatoes, peppers, onions, sweet basil, and oregano to make pasta sauce from scratch. There was even enough room to plant a small strawberry, blueberry, and raspberry patch so I could make homemade jams and desserts. And right in the center of it all was an already established robust Meyer lemon tree that I could envision leading to trays of fresh-from-the-oven lemon bars and pitchers of ice-cold lemonade.

Shortly before the wedding, I had secured a job as an executive assistant at a venture capital firm, mostly to help support us until Ryan passed the bar and I could chase my dream of being in PR or marketing in the city. But to be truthful, all I really wanted was to be a wife and mother. My dad always told Ryan that I wouldn't be happy until I was in the kitchen, an apron donning my waist, a baby clinging to my side, my foot closing the oven behind me, and a phone under my chin as I chatted to my mom or a girlfriend. I know it sounds old-fashioned, but that's what I really wanted—and now I had almost all of it. The only thing left was adding a baby to my hip.

Not long after we got back from our mini-moon, we received our photos from our wonderful wedding photographer, and Ryan and I laughed and reminisced as we went through them.

"Oh, look at this one," I said, pointing at us, two kids with our hands bound together and lifted triumphantly in the air as we walked out the chapel door toward our new life. "That's definitely my favorite one."

That's when I noticed it.

I had been feeling a little bloated the day of the wedding—that whole week, in fact. I'd even contemplated pulling on a pair of Spanx to help me get into my formfitting custom wedding gown. But I was already feeling cramped and uncomfortable, and I didn't want to make it even worse—especially with a full night of dancing ahead! And yet there it was, clear as day—to me anyway—a slight bump where there should have been smooth satin. *Hmmm* . . . , I thought, examining the picture a little more closely, *maybe I should have worn those Spanx. Amazing what stress can do to the body.* There was only one problem. The wedding was weeks ago. And yet my stomach was *still* bothering me.

"How long does the flu usually last?" I asked my mom the next time I talked with her. During the summer the doctor had diagnosed me with something called gastroenteritis, which sounded worse than the description I read online but felt different than the common flu. It was lingering.

"Why?" she asked. "Stomach still bothering you?"

"A little, yeah." I admitted. "I figured it was just a combination of the bug I had and all the pre-wedding stress, but it's been almost two months. I should be feeling better by now, wouldn't you think? I've barely gone to the bathroom, and I feel like I'm losing a lot of blood—and not the monthly kind."

"I'm sure it's nothing," she reassured me. "Maybe just hemorrhoids. If it's still bothering you in a couple of days, give your doctor a call."

The following weekend, Ryan and I were over at his parents' house watching a USC football game. When I stood up from the couch to help his mom bring in some snacks from the kitchen, I became so dizzy, I thought I was going to pass out. I steadied myself on the edge of the coffee table, but my head was spinning and I felt as though my legs would give out at any second. Something was definitely not right.

I sat back down next to Ryan. "Can I talk to you for a second?" I whispered in his ear. When he turned to look at me, his eyes grew wide.

"Wow. You're ghost-white. Are you okay?" he asked.

"I feel really weak and dizzy," I told him quietly, "and something's not right with my stomach."

I could read the concern on his face. "We're going to the ER."

I could only nod, hoping I wouldn't collapse from the dizziness or the cramps that had appeared out of nowhere. After standing back up, I leaned my hand against a wall to steady myself while Ryan made our excuses to his parents.

"Danielle isn't feeling well," he explained as casually as possible, "so we're going to take off."

I smiled weakly and leaned into Ryan for support. "Sorry," I offered, trying not to grimace. "Probably just a bug." No need whipping them into a panic—I was getting there quickly enough myself.

After assuring them we would call if we needed anything, Ryan ushered me to his car and took off toward the hospital. I leaned my head against the cool glass of the passenger side window and cradled my stomach. *Maybe I've got food poisoning*, I thought, quickly cataloging everything I'd eaten in the past twenty-four hours.

"Maybe it's food poisoning," Ryan echoed my thoughts. That almost made me laugh. Only eight weeks into our marriage, and we were already thinking alike.

"No," I shook my head. "You've eaten everything I have this week. If it were food poisoning, you'd have it too."

Ryan got quiet and gently rubbed my leg as I fought the urge to curl into the fetal position. Fortunately, the hospital was not far away, and within a matter of minutes, I found myself sitting on a cold ER exam table, shivering beneath a thin, gaping gown, hoping I wouldn't black out, throw up, or both before the doctor even had a chance to examine me.

Everything looked so sterile in the exam room—all metal, machines, and wires—not exactly a comforting environment. But at that moment, all I really cared about was making the pain go away.

After what felt like an eternity, the ER doctor came in, introduced himself, and asked what was going on with me.

I gave him a quick but thorough rundown of my symptoms, some of which I hadn't even told Ryan about—not because I was worried about frightening him, but because they were just plain embarrassing. What newlywed wants to hear about his blushing bride's infrequent bathroom visits? Or that what's coming out isn't looking like it should when it finally *does* come out?

One glance at Ryan told me he would have preferred to know—regardless.

"Let's run some tests to see what's going on," the doctor said when I was finished.

Ryan and I both nodded.

A few minutes later, a burly-looking man walked into my room and introduced himself as my nurse. "I'm here to draw some blood," he said. He put a rubber strap around my arm and pulled it tight to pop the vein. Then he ripped open a packet of sanitizer to sterilize my arm. The antiseptic chemical smell made me feel even more lightheaded.

"Make a fist," he said, then stuck in the needle. Four times. Ryan held my other hand, and I kept my eyes focused on him while this man attempted to successfully find a vein. I never look when I get my blood drawn. It just makes me queasy—or in this case, queasier.

After the blood draw, they performed a contrast dye CT scan, which basically involved injecting a dye into my body, which, when looked at on a monitor, would show them what was happening in my intestines. All I knew was that the dye filled my mouth with an awful metallic taste.

"At least they're being thorough," Ryan tried to reassure me. But with each test they ran, I became more and more anxious. *If they thought it was just the flu, they'd have given me a prescription for antibiotics and discharged me hours ago—like they did earlier this summer. What exactly are they trying to rule out? Or find?*

Finally, almost four hours later, just after one in the morning, the doctor came back with my results.

"Well, Ms. Walker," he began, flipping through the various lab results, "it appears that your colon is completely impacted from top to bottom. That's what's causing the intense cramping and likely the bleeding." He said it so matter-of-factly, as if this was a perfectly normal condition for an otherwise healthy twenty-two-year-old woman.

I looked over at Ryan. Of everything to get sick from, why did it have to be something so gross and embarrassing?

"So . . . what do we do now?" Ryan asked.

"I'm going to refer you to a gastroenterologist," he continued. "They specialize in treating the digestive system."

As the doctor wrote Ryan the referral, I sat stunned in my drafty gown. Aside from the occasional upset stomach as a child, I had always been perfectly healthy. And as far as I knew, nobody in my family had any history of digestive disorders. Four hours before, I'd come to the ER expecting them to give me a quick exam, tell me I had some hyperresistant strain of a flu bug, give me a shot and a prescription for antibiotics, and send me on my way. But now we were being referred to a specialist. *Specialists only see people who are seriously ill.* My mind raced, trying to think of anyone I'd ever known who had even *been* to a specialist, let alone been referred to one.

We probably should have asked more questions. *What does impaction mean? How do you fix it? Why did this happen? What other tests can we run to find out what is causing this?* But we were both exhausted and a little delirious, and at twenty-two, we had no understanding of how the body's intestines were supposed to function. So we walked out with only a fraction more information than we came in with. And a whole host of new questions that came to our minds as the shock and exhaustion turned to fear on the car ride home.

I'll just do some research on my laptop tomorrow after we get some rest, I thought to myself. Ryan hated when I did that. He always felt a professional opinion was best. I was a planner who hated surprises, so I figured I could educate myself on all the possibilities before we saw that gastro-whatever doctor. At least then I could start to prepare for the worst and hope for the best.

3

With slightly shaking hands and a nervous lump in my throat, I called the gastrointestinal doctor first thing the next morning.

"I'm sorry, he's booked with other patients for the next two weeks," his receptionist told me.

I tried to explain my situation, hoping that *somehow* she would squeeze me into his schedule. She just repeated herself and asked if I wanted to book an appointment for two weeks from that day.

What choice do I have? I thought. As I waited to see the doctor, I was often in tears because I was in so much pain and exhausted from what I was experiencing—or more accurately, what I *wasn't* experiencing.

Meanwhile, I spent countless hours and many late nights researching every health and medical site I could find online that appeared legit, only to disappear down one rabbit hole after another. With each encouraging bit I read, I breathed a sigh of relief. *Oh good, it's just that some people aren't as regular as others* and *I'll eventually go back to normal*. But then I'd stumble upon something frightening that made my symptoms appear life-threatening. And the more I read, the more terrifying everything became.

"Ryan!" I yelled one night as I stared at my laptop, the blue light from the screen illuminating the tears rolling down my cheeks. "Come here, quick!"

"What?" Ryan said, rushing into the room, eyes wide in alarm.

"I have colon cancer!" I could barely get the words out; I was nearly hyperventilating.

"What?" he repeated, this time in confusion.

"Listen to this," I told him and began to blurt out all the cancer symptoms listed. "'A persistent change in your bowel habits, including . . . constipation. . . . blood in your stool. Persistent abdominal discomfort, such as cramps, gas or pain. A feeling that your bowel doesn't empty completely. Weakness or fatigue.' I match *all* of these!" I hiccupped with the tears that were now coming fast and furious. "And this other article says that the number of young adults getting colon cancer is going way up!" I looked into his eyes, petrified.

Ryan sat beside me and squeezed my hand. "Danielle, please stop reading that stuff. It's freaking you out and probably doesn't even pertain to you. Let's not jump to conclusions," he said calmly, rubbing my back. "Let's just wait to see what the specialist says, okay?"

I tried to inhale slowly to get myself under control and then nodded. That would be the first of many times Ryan would be my voice of reason. My stabilizer. My advocate. I hoped desperately he was right. But something nagged at me. Whatever was happening didn't feel right, and it clearly wasn't going away.

When the day of my appointment finally came, Ryan insisted on going with me, and honestly, I was grateful. Two weeks of self-diagnosing online had only heightened my sense of panic. At least one of us needed to remain calm and coherent enough to process whatever this guy had to say.

"Mr. and Mrs. Walker," the specialist greeted us in the exam room, "I'm Dr. Kendhari." He was an older gentleman, probably in his mid- to late sixties, with an olive complexion and glasses, wearing the requisite white lab coat.

"Let's see what we have here." As he flipped through the test results the ER had forwarded, I glanced nervously around the room. The walls were covered in illustrations of the stomach and intestines. I flashed back to the CT scan they took in the ER and wondered how my insides compared to the ones on the walls.

Finally I couldn't stand the silence anymore. "Is there any chance I have colon cancer?" I nearly choked on the words, terrified that he'd say yes.

"Yes, there could be a very small chance that you have colon cancer," he said casually, his eyes never leaving my file.

My chest and throat both constricted. I couldn't breathe. I squeezed Ryan's hand so tight that his fingertips turned purple.

"But more likely," he continued, "you're just constipated and need more fiber in your diet. I wouldn't worry too much about it." He looked up at me and smiled.

My mind was racing to comprehend not only what he said, but what he *hadn't* said. *He didn't say it wasn't cancer. Is he just ruling that out? What if he's wrong? What if I do have cancer? What if . . .* Before I could even articulate a response, he continued.

"I'd suggest wheat bran. Start putting a full cup of it into a smoothie every day. And pick up some MiraLAX. You can get it at any grocery store. I'll also give you some enemas that you can administer to help move things along."

I was still struggling to wrap my head around what he was telling me when he closed my file and said, "That should take care of it. Give my office a call if you need anything else." And with that he politely shook Ryan's hand and walked out of the room.

That's it? Eat more fiber? He didn't even examine me. Or ask if I had any questions. Or rule out colon cancer! I wasn't sure what tests there were to look into things like this, but surely there had to be *something* else to check.

I looked over at Ryan. "I thought he'd run other tests—stuff the ER couldn't do. Isn't that the whole point of seeing a specialist?"

Ryan just shook his head, his mouth hanging open in disbelief. "I guess he feels it's not that serious. That's a good thing, though, right?"

I supposed he had a point. After all, this guy was a specialist. He dealt with this kind of thing—and presumably much worse—all the time. Maybe it *was* good that he felt whatever I had could be treated at home with an extra scoop of fiber a day. Still, I'd expected . . . more.

On the way home, Ryan and I stopped at a health-food store, where I bought a large container of dusty, flaky wheat bran, and our local drugstore, where I picked up a big purple bottle of MiraLAX, clinging to the hope that I *was* just constipated and not cancer-ridden. All the while, one simple question kept ringing in my head—the one I couldn't seem to articulate in the ER or the gastroenterologist's office—*Why?* I no longer believed these were just the side effects of being stressed over the wedding or the move. I'd been stressed plenty of times before and *never* had this kind of reaction. And even though it was a stomach issue, I couldn't think of anything different or unusual I'd eaten over the past several months that could have led to this. There just didn't seem to be any rhyme or reason to it. I knew something was seriously off. But if even the specialist wasn't concerned . . . maybe I was overreacting.

As soon as we got home, I pulled out our new blender, a wedding present from one of my cousins, and filled it with a full cup of bran, plus the MiraLAX, yogurt, and frozen berries. I didn't know how it would taste. After all, I'd never mixed a cup of fiber into anything before, so I just gulped the smoothie down as quickly as possible. Normally, I loved smoothies; the sweet and creamy flavors filled me up and gave me energy throughout the day. This, however, tasted sludgy, earthy, and, frankly, terrible. But that wasn't the worst of it.

From all my midnight internet research, I knew that insoluble fiber from foods like wheat bran, whole grains, and cereals could help everything move more quickly through the intestines. What I didn't know was that when someone is already fully impacted, those high-fiber foods have nowhere to go. Instead, they just add more pressure and substance to everything that is already backed up, making the condition even worse.

As for the enemas? *Did the person who wrote the instructions with the little cartoon person lying calmly on their side with one leg strewn over the other realize just how impossible it is for said person to reach around their own body and squeeze a bottle of liquid up their own behind?* I wondered. *No, I'm sure they did not.*

The other part they left out of the instructions was, "Ask your newlywed husband to do it for you."

"For better or worse, in sickness and in health?" I said to Ryan in a lighthearted tone that felt like anything but a joke as I handed him the squeeze bottle.

My poor, sweet husband. He was so calm, nonjudgmental, and caring. Still, I couldn't imagine a worse nightmare for a newlywed.

Day after day, I continued to down wheat bran and MiraLAX like candy, and by the fourth day, the pain was crippling. It felt as though someone had put a balloon into my colon and overinflated it to the point that it could burst at any minute.

"Maybe you should stop," Ryan suggested.

"The MiraLAX bottle says to use it for up to seven days," I said, reviewing the dosage instructions. "Maybe it just takes time to go into effect."

"Maybe we should get a second opinion," Ryan countered.

I hadn't even considered that possibility, but given that things weren't improving, and in fact, were getting worse, I was inclined to agree. But who? What makes one gastroenterologist better than another? How are you supposed to research a specialist when you're not even sure what's wrong with you?

The next morning while Ryan was at school, I started calling around to other GI specialists in the area, but everyone I called was either not accepting new patients or was booked for weeks.

Then one night my dad called. "I got you an appointment," he said, the concern in his voice evident. "I asked a friend who manages hospitals to recommend a GI specialist. This doctor is really good, and he is willing to see you."

Two days later, Ryan and I found ourselves sitting in yet another exam room. I could tell instantly that Dr. Beale was different. He was kind and sensitive, and instead of just reading my files, he sat down and took the time to talk to me.

"Tell me about your symptoms," he said, looking me in the eye as though he had no other patient except me.

I told him about the cramps, the bleeding, the dizziness, and all the fiber I had been trying to consume. He nodded sympathetically. Then he looked over the test results and scans, and said, "They shouldn't have had you taking all that. You're so severely impacted that there's nowhere for everything to go."

I glanced at Ryan and could tell he was thinking the same thing I was. *How could the other specialist not have known that?*

"Given that your colon is still impacted," he continued, "and your bleeding has not yet subsided, I'd like to admit you to the hospital. In fact, I'd like you to go there immediately."

My stomach clenched, not from the cramps but from escalating fear. Aside from a broken arm from performing too many back walkovers on the pavement when I was ten, the only other time I'd even been to the ER was when this whole thing began. And I had never been *admitted* to a hospital before.

"Can I go home first to pack up some things and take care of loose ends?" I asked.

He shook his head. "I strongly advise against it. You need to get in there now." Though his voice remained calm, there was no mistaking the seriousness of his tone. I wasn't sure if I should be afraid or relieved. On the one hand, someone was finally taking my symptoms as seriously as I was. But when a specialist basically orders you to get to a hospital immediately, how can you not start to panic just a little?

"This is actually good," Ryan assured me as we walked across the parking lot from the medical building to the hospital. "Dr. Beale seems to know what he's talking about. At least now you'll get some real treatment."

"I hope so," I said, squeezing his hand tighter.

Once I got settled into my room, Ryan ran back to the house to pick up some of my things. I did my best to keep my mind off the worst-case scenarios, but the only question that kept running through my mind was *Am I going to die?* The fact that the receptionist downstairs had walked us through a living will as we filled out the other paperwork certainly hadn't helped.

I can't die—I just got married. I still have my whole life ahead of me.

I was so relieved when Ryan returned. Just having him there calmed me down a little.

"We're going to figure this out—together—okay?" he said, holding both of my hands in his. "We're a team. We'll get through this. 'For better or for worse,' remember?" His unwavering belief that everything was going to turn out okay gave me strength.

Thirty-six hours later, after a horrifying prep process and colonoscopy, Dr. Beale came into my room to give us the results.

"Your results are slightly inconclusive," he said. "But you don't have cancer."

Ryan and I both breathed a massive sigh of relief.

"It looks like you have a severe case of ulcerative colitis, but it could be Crohn's disease. We need to wait for biopsies to come back."

I shifted uncomfortably in my bed and racked my brain for where I'd heard the term *ulcerative colitis* before. I knew I'd run across it in my extensive online research, but I couldn't remember much about it.

"Ulcerative colitis is similar to Crohn's disease, but they affect different parts of the intestinal tract," he explained. "Basically, it means that your entire colon is inflamed and filled with open wounds and scar tissue."

So many questions ran through my mind—but I could articulate none of them.

"The good news is, there are medications for it," he continued.

"Great," I said, smiling for the first time in what felt like days. "How long do I have to take them before I'm back to normal?"

His smile faded, and his eyebrows furrowed in concern. "Danielle, this isn't a curable condition. You'll have it for life."

For life. That completely knocked the wind out of me. My mind raced. "Can I . . . can *we* still have kids?" I was almost afraid to look at Ryan.

A gentle smile returned to the doctor's face. "Yes, you can have a regular life. The medications will allow you to live normally and won't interfere with a pregnancy."

I heard the air rush out of my lungs in a jagged sigh of relief. "Okay," I smiled up at Ryan. *This is just a setback.* I leaned back against my pillow, my muscles slowly beginning to relax. *The medication will take care of everything, and my life will go back to normal.*

"What caused this?" Ryan asked. While I was glad he thought to ask, at that moment I wasn't all that concerned with the cause. I just wanted to know how to get rid of it.

Dr. Beale shrugged slightly. "We don't really know. It could be hereditary, it could be stress, but it can also just appear out of nowhere."

"Do I still need to take the MiraLAX and wheat bran?" I asked.

"No, the impaction you're experiencing isn't typical with this kind of disease. In fact, it's usually the other way around. So I'm going to recommend that you stop taking those."

"Is there anything I *should* do?" I asked. "Anything I should eat or not eat or . . . ?"

He shook his head. "Diet doesn't cause it, can't cure it, and won't help it. You can, however, steer clear—for the time being—of anything raw, like salads, vegetables, and fruits. Those can be really tough on your system, especially right now, after what you've just gone through. You can also follow the low-residue diet," he continued, "which is essentially nothing high fiber. No whole grains or cereals, nuts, seeds. Try to eat foods that have refined or enriched grains, such as white flour, white sugar, white pasta, and white rice. You can have limited fruit, but avoid the skins and seeds."

That sounded easy enough. I was already eating all those things!

"But really I wouldn't worry so much about what you eat," he added. "The medications I'm going to give you will take care of everything."

"Thank you, Dr. Beale," Ryan said gratefully.

"You're welcome," he said, smiling. "Let me get a prescription written up for you, and then you should be able to go home today."

A few hours later, I was discharged from the hospital with prescriptions for a steroid called prednisone to help control the inflammation and suppress the immune system, an anti-inflammatory called mesalamine that I was told was like a slow-releasing Advil for my colon, and suppositories to decrease the bleeding, swelling, and irritation.

The next day, I felt a little better, though I still didn't have all my strength back. I took a few sick days so I could rest and try to get a handle on my newly diagnosed health issue. Ryan had warned me not to spend any more time researching my symptoms online, but it bugged me that I'd gone through all that hassle at the hospital and really only learned the name of what I had. No one explained what ulcerative colitis was, what I should expect from it, and what it meant for the rest of my life. I was just given a few prescriptions and the assurance that I would be fine.

But I had the nagging feeling that there might be more to it, and besides the prescriptions, the doctor had released me from the hospital without providing so much as a pamphlet on what this disease actually was. I felt like I knew no more than when I was admitted—other than a name to associate my symptoms with.

So while Ryan was at class, I started doing a little digging on my laptop.

One of my go-to sources for medical information was the Mayo Clinic, so I looked up their page on inflammatory bowel disease first. It explained that ulcerative colitis (or UC) "involves inflammation and sores (ulcers) along the superficial lining of your large intestine (colon) and rectum." Symptoms include "diarrhea, rectal bleeding, abdominal pain, fatigue and weight loss."

It sounded awful. *But the medicine will make me feel better,* I assured myself.

And it did . . . for a while. My symptoms slowly began to lessen, but then different issues began to arise. Within a few weeks of taking the drugs, my cheeks swelled up like a puffer fish. It wasn't painful, but as a young newlywed, it did make me feel incredibly self-conscious. And I was hungry *all the time*. I ate six to eight meals a day and still wanted more, yet I wasn't gaining any weight, which seemed weird.

But the worst was the insomnia. While Ryan slept peacefully, I'd lie wide-awake. Frustrated, I'd usually pull myself out of bed, wander into the living room, plop down on the couch, and channel surf.

I found myself watching the Cartoon Network or infomercials until four in the morning, and I had to be energized and ready to go to work by 8:00 a.m. It was a vicious cycle that left me drained, and to be honest, a little cranky.

Then the mood swings hit. All my emotions seemed magnified and hyped up. I could be fine one minute and then, as if a light switch flipped on inside, I became furious or weepy, which was totally out of character for me. The only good side effect was that I became so neurotic that I cleaned every inch of my house during my energy bursts. We're talking toothpicks-in-cracks clean.

Wondering whether these were, in fact, side effects, I grabbed my laptop and began to do a little more research. I typed in *ulcerative colitis* and found very little information on how to treat it, other than with the medications I was already on. But I was relieved to learn that at least I wasn't alone in what I was experiencing. One source I found said that well over one million people in the United States suffer from inflammatory bowel diseases. It also said that the best treatment was the medicine I was taking. In fact, according to that source, in 2004, 2.1 million prescriptions were written for medications to treat what I had.

Then I looked up the possible side effects of the medicines I was taking. The list was longer than my arm: hiccups, weight gain, high blood pressure, headaches, muscle weakness, nausea, vomiting, thinning skin, restlessness, insomnia, puffiness of the face (moon face), growth of facial hair, easy bruising of the skin, impaired wound healing, glaucoma, cataracts, ulcers, irregular periods, seizures, hives, skin rashes, vision changes, diabetes, congestive heart failure, heart attacks, pulmonary edema, hyperglycemia, hypothyroidism, anemia, amnesia, depression, extreme mood swings, psychotic behavior, personality changes, osteonecrosis . . . The list went on and on. *Oh my gosh*, I thought. *The cure is almost worse than the disease!*

"I don't like what's happening to me," I told Ryan one morning after another night without sleep. I grabbed a muffin and swallowed it with my morning coffee. "I'm not myself. I feel like I'm—" I paused, hating to say it aloud—"going crazy."

"Maybe it's because you haven't been sleeping?" he offered.

"Maybe. But it seems like more than that. Something's off. I've never felt this way before. And I don't think it's the UC."

Ryan nodded. "Okay, let's call the doctor and see what he has to say."

Dr. Beale didn't seem too concerned. "You don't need to worry about those side effects. They'll go away as soon as we wean you off the prednisone." He also prescribed Ambien to help me sleep.

I awoke the next morning having slept but not feeling refreshed. And all the weirdness returned in full. My brain felt off, as though I was in my body but out of it. If the prednisone had side effects, I wondered if Ambien did as well, so I looked them up. Sure enough: decreased awareness, hallucinations, changes in behavior, memory problems, sleepwalking, drowsiness, dizziness, grogginess, feeling as if you have been drugged—even diarrhea and insomnia. I definitely did not need more of those!

Is this the "normal" I have to look forward to for the rest of my life? I was glad my colon had calmed down, but I wasn't so sure the solution was much better. *No, Danielle, just suck it up. This will last only a little while, then I'll be off the medicine and I'll be all good again.*

At least my UC symptoms seemed to be under control, just as Dr. Beale predicted, which was good because Thanksgiving was approaching, and Ryan and I were going to host this year's feast.

Our whole family had been invited to our modest and cozy duplex—Ryan's parents, my parents, both of my siblings and their spouses, and my grandparents. I wasn't sure how I was going to squeeze twelve adults in, but I figured it would work out somehow.

———————————

"Are you sure you're up for it?" my mom asked when I called to get her advice on cooking the twenty-pound bird. "It's a lot of work. And with you just getting out of the hospital?"

"Yes, I'm sure," I reassured her. "This is something I really want to do." I had waited my entire life to host this kind of gathering—to create memories; to share life, love, and laughter; to enjoy board games, delicious food, and a friendly game of flag football together. There was no way I was going to allow puffy cheeks and UC to stand in my way—especially after all Ryan and I had been through the previous months. Now, more than ever, I recognized how much I had to truly be grateful for, and I wanted to share that with my loved ones.

The one real challenge to making the day a success was the turkey. I had never cooked one before. But I remembered my mom putting a Butterball into a big plastic bag and hours later pulling out a perfectly cooked bird, ready to slice. *It can't be that difficult.* But then visions of serving that raw chicken Parmesan to Ryan and his roommates quickly sprang to mind. *No way. This is going to be perfect.*

The next morning, I was up bright and early to get the bird prepared and in the oven so it would be ready in time for dinner. My mom came over to help.

"Did you rinse it really well, both outside and inside?" she asked.

"Um . . . yeah," I said, even though I couldn't remember rinsing the inside of it.

"Where's the bag of giblets and the neck?" Mom asked, looking around the counters and in the sink.

"What bag of giblets?" I stared blankly at her.

"From inside the turkey. There's a little bag inside the cavity. It contains the heart, liver, and gizzard. The neck is in there as well. You would have felt them when you rinsed it."

We both looked at the oven.

"You didn't take it out?"

I shook my head. "Is that bad?"

She laughed. "Well, we'll see. We can't take it out now because we've sealed up the baking bag."

When the turkey was finally cooked, I took it out of the baking bag, separated the legs, reached in with tongs and pulled out a shriveled-up bag filled with off-color, hardened body parts. The oven had a faint smell of melted plastic, but the bird looked intact.

"What am I supposed to do with these?"

"Well normally, you use them to make broth for the gravy that simmers while the turkey cooks," my mom said, laughing again.

My dad and Grandma Marge were always the gravy makers. So once Grandma Marge arrived and had a good chuckle over my turkey story, I listened as she gave me directions. She had me use cornstarch whisked with a little water to make a "slurry," a packet of powdered gravy as starter, Kitchen Bouquet to make it a deeper brown, and lots of salt and pepper. Then she had me take that slurry and mix it into the pan drippings to thicken it up.

My mom was right; Thanksgiving dinner was a big undertaking, and nowhere near as simple as I'd thought it was, growing up. Besides making the box of Stove Top Stuffing and occasionally helping with the mashed potatoes, the three of us kids would just appear in our Sunday best at the table on Thanksgiving evening after my mom had lined up everything on the counter. We eventually added the creamy green bean casserole to our list of contributions, but I had no idea how much work went into it all.

When the guests began to arrive, each with their assigned side dishes, I breathed a sigh of relief. Grandma Marge may have refused a potluck meal, but I certainly wasn't going to! *Who in their right mind makes upwards of twelve dishes in one day?*

When we added the leaf to our new dining table from the Crate and Barrel outlet (which we'd used the last of our wedding gift cards to buy), it filled the entire dining room, and we were barely able to pull the chairs out without hitting the walls. It was cramped, but all that mattered was that the house was filled with the people we loved.

After we prayed a blessing over our meal and our family, we piled our plates high. I threw all the low-residue stuff out the window for this meal and ate all of our family classics: mashed potatoes topped with that semi-homemade gravy, green bean casserole covered in cream of mushroom soup and topped with French's fried onions, sweet potatoes slathered in brown sugar with marshmallow topping, Hawaiian sweet rolls, jiggly cranberry sauce (still in that cylindrical shape with the ridges from the can), store-bought Stove Top Stuffing with the packet of spices and a blob of butter, the richest pumpkin and pecan pies with mounds of whipped cream, and of course the turkey, which everybody complimented me on.

After our final guests left, I plopped down next to Ryan on the couch, exhausted but happy. "We did it, babe," I sighed contentedly. And the turkey didn't smell or taste like burnt plastic! This was the life I had imagined and looked forward to since I was a little girl. And for all my frustrations with the medicine, it seemed to be doing its job.

Finally, everything was starting to feel normal.

4

By the following March I felt much better, and I was determined to get off the steroids. I just couldn't take what they were doing to me any longer, so at my next doctor's appointment I presented my case to Dr. Beale.

"We can wean you off of them," he conceded, "but you can't quit cold turkey." I knew that was true because I'd thoroughly studied the list of side effects and warnings about discontinuing prednisone all at once. In fact, stopping looked almost as scary as staying on it.

"Fine. I just want to get off them as quickly and as safely as I can."

Dr. Beale set a schedule for leveling out the dosages over the next two months—perfect timing because that June my work colleagues, parents, siblings and their spouses, Ryan, and I would be going on a humanitarian trip to Africa.

The company I worked for had a family foundation that sponsored a water filtration project in camps for refugees and internally displaced persons (IDP) in northern Uganda, along the border of South Sudan, and they wanted to check on its progress. Twenty-five people were going, and I was in charge of planning all the logistics for our fifteen-day trip. I'd booked the flights, hotels, and transportation, and I'd arranged all the meals.

A month before we left, we had to get a litany of vaccinations that the United States required for us to travel to Uganda, including shots for hepatitis A and B, typhoid fever, and meningitis, along with booster shots for measles/mumps/rubella, polio, and tetanus. We also were given malaria pills and an antibiotic pack to have on hand in case anyone got traveler's diarrhea.

A week or so after the vaccinations, I started to notice uncomfortable gut symptoms again but figured it was just a combination of my body being worn down from the stress of handling the last-minute details and readjusting after weaning off the prednisone.

Then about a week before our departure, my symptoms escalated. I was losing blood and couldn't leave the house. Then came the pain and cramping. It never crossed my mind that the vaccinations could have stirred something up until my brother-in-law, Tyson, who had a mild case of UC himself, mentioned he was having symptoms after getting the shots.

I immediately called Dr. Beale. "We've got this trip to Uganda planned, and I'm starting to have symptoms." I paused, feeling almost like I was a little girl asking my dad to let me go to a party. "Do you think it's safe for me to go?" *Please say yes.*

It was his turn to pause for a moment. Then he asked me a series of questions about frequency, urgency, pain, and bleeding. "Yes," he finally said. "I think it's fine for you to go. Although I'd feel better about your trip if you would get back on the prednisone. We'll put you on a lower dose so you shouldn't have such intense side effects, okay?"

Reluctantly, I started back on a low-dose regime of twenty

milligrams of prednisone, willing it to take care of the UC and not make me feel as crazy as it had before.

As our departure date drew nearer, I took notice of how I felt. On the days I felt normal, I would announce to Ryan, "I feel good today. I'm going to be okay. The medicine is managing it." But then a couple of days later, I would regress and not feel well. "We probably shouldn't go," I'd say sadly. The almost-daily mental tug-of-war between the decision to go or to stay home was exhausting and maddening. We spent a lot of time praying for wisdom about it, and Ryan and I encouraged each other by saying, "If God wants us to go, he'll protect us."

The night before our trip was miserable. I was up practically all night going in and out of the bathroom, and I started to feel dizzy again. Maybe it was the lack of sleep and the turmoil from going back and forth on our decision, but I was restless, and my nerves were on high alert.

"Honey, I know we really want to go," Ryan said, "but are you sure you want to be in a place that's so far from your doctor and where we have no idea what the doctors and medical situation are like? Maybe we should just stay home."

With tears in my eyes, I slowly nodded, but I still wasn't committed to canceling. It wasn't just that I had worked so hard to help put the trip together; I really believed in what we were going to do there. I felt deeply for those who were suffering and needed something as simple and life-giving as clean water. I wanted to love on the beautiful, innocent children who had been forced to suffer from the untold trauma that had brought them to those camps.

As I lay on the couch in pain and desperation, we prayed that if God wanted us to go, he would show us by helping me feel better through the night.

The following morning, I felt good. I had energy, and I wasn't in pain. I was convinced the worst was behind me and the medication had finally kicked in—providing that "normal" life I had been promised.

"Okay, let's do this. Let's go," I told Ryan as I pulled out my traveling clothes and started to put them on.

Ryan's eyes widened. "Are you *sure*?"

"Absolutely. I need to do this. Plus, I don't want you to miss this trip because of me. The doctor said it was all clear; we've been praying about it. I'm sure I'll be fine." *And even if I'm not,* I figured, *I have my medicine. We can always call Dr. Beale if anything goes wrong.*

The next day, Ryan and I pulled up to my parents' house to board the black twenty-passenger bus I'd reserved, poised to take off for the airport. The looks my parents, siblings, and their spouses gave me said what their mouths couldn't—they were afraid for me.

C'mon, guys, I wanted to say. *What have we always talked about? That if we pray and believe, we'll receive the desires of our heart.*

I smiled, hoping that would put everyone at ease. After we all piled into the bus, I buckled my seat belt and sat back. Ryan took my hand and gave it a squeeze of reassurance, but I didn't miss the concern in his eyes. He, too, wondered whether we were making the right decision. I squeezed back and smiled.

"I'll be fine," I assured him. "Don't worry."

The six-hour flight from San Francisco to New York was uneventful—until the descent. I began to feel the rumblings of nausea and abdominal cramping coming on as the pressure changed in the cabin.

"Oof," I grimaced, clutching my stomach.

"You okay?" Even though I had tried to keep quiet, Ryan still noticed.

I swallowed hard and through gritted teeth told him yes. *Hold on, just hold on,* I told myself.

After disembarking in New York, we boarded the enormous transatlantic jet that would take us on the next leg of our journey—all the way to Dubai in the United Arab Emirates. We would stay there for a night before continuing. I glanced at my ticket to see my seat assignment. Dead center in a long, six-seat row of strangers. Holding on to my carry-on with one hand and my stomach with the other, I squeezed by the passengers sharing my row. The pain in my abdomen intensified, and the scent of food mixed with various bodily scents around me didn't help. As others looked for the exit doors in case of an emergency, I scanned for the nearest restrooms. They already had a line. Panic began to build.

A kind-looking, fresh-faced flight attendant stopped by and asked about our group. When one of our team explained that we were headed to Uganda for humanitarian efforts, she smiled brightly. Then she noticed me. My face must have been broadcasting my pain and fragility. Her face drew dark with concern, and she walked away quickly. Within a few moments, she reappeared.

"Why don't you come with me?" she said. "And bring your carry-on."

Confused, I looked at Ryan, who shrugged and nodded his encouragement. I did as she asked and followed her toward the front of the plane, past row after row of economy seating. When we moved into the business-class section, my jaw dropped. *How is this possible?*

She stopped at one of the empty and quite roomy, comfortable-looking seats. "Here you go." She stepped aside for me to sit. "It reclines better than the ones back there." She jutted her chin toward the back of the plane, toward my old seat. "This also has a designated restroom that only the twenty passengers in this section can use."

"Thank you," I said, genuinely gushing over her kindness and trying not to cry.

Even in business class, with a comfy seat and lots of room to spread out, the nearly fifteen-hour voyage was more than my body could handle. I situated and resituated my body to get as comfortable as possible, but nothing seemed to alleviate the pressure. The pain I'd hoped would disappear from sheer willpower and the renewed dose of prednisone failed to dissipate. It felt as though my insides were rolling around an unending minefield.

It's just because of the cabin pressure, I reasoned with myself. *Once we land, I'll stretch out in a nice, comfortable bed and sleep. That will do the trick. It's just the stress of travel. This won't last.*

After leaving Dubai, we made a brief tarmac stop in Addis Ababa, Ethiopia. After that, we finally landed in Entebbe, Uganda, nearly forty-eight hours after departing San Francisco.

We then made the thirty-mile drive to Kampala, our final destination. The roads we took to get there were like nothing I had ever seen—far different even from the streets and poverty I had witnessed in Juarez, Mexico, as a teen on a mission trip. Motorbikes packed tightly with two or even three passengers weaved recklessly between gridlocked cars, some of them going against traffic just to get somewhere faster. Pedestrians walked between cars, going any direction they chose and claiming the right-of-way.

Once we got out of the city, the drive became even more treacherous, and with every bump I thought I was going to pass out from the pain. We waited on the less-congested roads as goats and cows slowly traipsed from one side to the other. I wasn't expecting the shantytowns—a stark difference from the high-rises and flats we'd seen in the city center. My heart broke to see slabs of cardboard propped up to form makeshift homes. Children peeked their heads out from behind clothes blowing in the wind that had been hung on lines to dry and waved in excitement as they saw the car drive by.

Those were the little faces I was looking forward to serving and singing lullabies to; the little bodies I was looking forward to holding tight and swinging around in the air until they were laughing and so dizzy they could barely walk a straight line. Those were the children

I wanted to teach silly American songs to; the babies I wanted to snuggle to give their exhausted mothers a rest.

I clutched my churning stomach as another wave of nausea washed over me and cramps constricted my abdomen.

"Are you okay?" Ryan leaned in, his face a mask of concern.

I took a deep breath and slowly let it out, trying—and failing—to regain control of my system. He was so close I barely had to turn my head to look right into his eyes, and I was grateful because I didn't want to panic the others. Fighting back tears, I whispered, "I think we might have made a mistake." We were clearly a world away from the comforts of home, and all I wanted was my own bed and close proximity to my doctor.

Ryan and I spent our first night in Uganda with me locked away in our hotel bathroom in excruciating pain, vomiting violently for hours on end. When we tried calling Dr. Beale, his service informed us that he was on vacation. That left us only one option: a small Ugandan hospital located roughly three miles from our hotel.

My dad and Ryan called for a cab and rode there with me. After a fifteen-minute drive, we stopped in front of a single-story, dingy-white dilapidated building that looked as if it hadn't seen paint or a hammer in decades. An old van that had been made into an ambulance sat in front with the words *The Surgery* painted on it in royal blue. I swallowed hard and thought seriously about telling the cab driver to take us back to the hotel.

"I'm sure it's not as bad as it looks," Ryan assured me. My dad, on the other hand, looked dubious. And candidly, I was with *him*.

We entered the two-room building, and a kind nurse greeted us and escorted me to an old discolored white plastic lawn chair. *If the blood draw chair looks like this, what condition will the needles be in?* I breathed a sigh of relief when I watched the nurse rip open a sanitary package and withdraw a sharp needle. She wiped down my arm with an alcohol swab, wrapped a plastic tie around my arm, had me make a fist, and tapped the inside of my arm to find a good vein from which to draw blood. *Okay . . . so far so good.*

I looked around the makeshift hospital. The beds were wooden planks with paper-thin mats placed on top—no box springs or mattresses—and bugs were crawling everywhere. *Maybe we should go . . .* , I thought to myself. But before I could express my concerns to Ryan, a tall, distinguished-looking, gray-haired man appeared in the doorway.

"Mrs. Walker?" he said, smiling. "I'm Dr. Stark." He had a British accent that I found strangely comforting. "I'm afraid you are severely anemic and dehydrated." That was less comforting. He paused and looked at me with compassion in his eyes. "You are having a serious flare-up. I'm afraid you're in critical condition." He paused again to let the severity of his diagnosis sink in.

As Ryan, my dad, and I exchanged concerned glances, Dr. Stark scanned my blood test results. "I have never seen such high levels of inflammation coupled with such acute anemia and dehydration. Nor have I ever seen this severe a case of an autoimmune disease."

His words swirled around my mind as I tried to take it all in. I was in a strange hospital in a developing country, and I had just been told I had an *autoimmune disease*—a term no other doctor had used to describe my condition before. I wasn't even sure what that meant, but paired with *critical condition*, it didn't take much of a leap to figure out it wasn't good.

"I'm sorry," my dad broke in. "What exactly does all of that mean?"

"The anemia," Dr. Stark explained, "is from blood loss. The dehydration is probably a result of excessive vomiting and diarrhea. You're eating, but your gut isn't able to absorb the nutrients your body needs. It's all seeping out. That is one of the challenges of your particular autoimmune disease. In Uganda, where we tragically experience a multitude of other ailments and diseases, we rarely if ever see autoimmune diseases."

"Why is that?" Ryan asked.

"Perhaps it's because this country isn't overly sterile, like the US and other westernized nations," he suggested. "The children here grow up with the understanding that God made dirt, and dirt doesn't hurt. They play in it. They eat from it. They likely have parasites, but they aren't given antibiotics from birth for a simple ear infection, for instance. They aren't usually born by cesarean, which increases the risk of autoimmune conditions and allergies from the start due to the antibiotics administered to the mother and the lack of beneficial flora passed to the infant during a vaginal birth."

I thought about the hand sanitizers and bleach wipes I'd been instructed to bring with me and had already used dozens of times since boarding the first flight in San Francisco. We'd been lectured before we left the States to wash our hands frequently and not drink the water or eat any raw food because the parasites would make us sick. Along with our vaccinations, we'd even been given a ready-to-pop Z-Pak in case any of that happened. This antibiotic, azithromycin, would completely wipe out the bacteria—both good and bad—just as the ones I'd been administered before my colonoscopy had.

"Everything in the US is bleached and overly cleaned," he continued. "As soon as your kids drop something on the floor, you're wiping it down with sterilized towelettes. You have an overly sanitized nation, and as a result, many of you have an overgrowth of unhealthy bacteria and an underrepresentation of healthy bacteria in your gut." He looked at me. "And in some cases, that can contribute to autoimmune diseases like Crohn's disease, UC, rheumatoid arthritis, and a host of others. The people here eat their food fresh from the ground. Most don't wash their hands before eating, and they don't always use silverware. They eat the things they have grown without washing them, so their food has natural microorganisms on it. They're not bleaching it or spraying it with something to kill all the bacteria."

"If nobody here has this disease because of the way they eat and prepare their food," I said, clutching my still-churning stomach, "then why don't we do it that way at home?"

He explained that in America, we tend to go for immediate gratification—whatever's quickest and most convenient. That means the food we are growing is often altered to grow faster. By using genetically modified (GMO) seeds, pesticides, and insecticides, growers also produce crops that are less susceptible to damage.

Not only has much of our food been altered from the way God intended it and the way it *used to be* grown, but we, as a culture, have moved far from the practices of our grandmothers and great-grandmothers, who cooked from scratch using unprocessed foods. Half the ingredients listed on the prepackaged items most of us eat today are barely even pronounceable. They aren't found in nature. We created them to make "real food" look nicer and last longer.

In addition, we wash and bleach fruits and vegetables to the point that virtually none of the natural, healthy bacteria or probiotics from the soil are left on them. To top it off, we pick food early—before it's fully ripe—so it can be transported to grocery stores, some of which spray the produce with even more chemicals to slow the ripening process.

We're also one of the only cultures that doesn't regularly incorporate natural forms of fermented foods like sauerkraut, kimchi, and kefir into our diet—natural probiotics that add beneficial bacteria and enzymes to our intestinal flora, increase the health of our gut and digestive system, and enhance the immune system. The less diverse our gut flora, the higher the risk of chronic inflammatory conditions such as inflammatory bowel disease, Crohn's, and UC.

Had I not been in so much pain and so utterly exhausted from the travel and lack of sleep, I could have listened to Dr. Stark talk for hours. After consulting with two GI specialists and undergoing a battery of scans, biopsies, and blood tests in some of the most sophisticated medical facilities in the Bay Area, who would have guessed that the most thorough explanation of what I had and how I might have gotten it would come from a doctor in a dilapidated two-room hospital in the middle of a developing country. I still believed God wanted me to come to Uganda. Now I was starting to wonder if maybe he had brought me here so I could start to learn how to help my body heal itself.

Diet doesn't cause it. Diet won't help it. Diet can't cure it. Every single one of the doctors I had seen before now had rattled off that same narrative. But Dr. Stark had such a different opinion. Who was correct? And if the gut bacteria that Dr. Stark was talking about was so important, why didn't my doctors have me take probiotics after my colonoscopy or after I'd taken all the antibiotics they'd prescribed me?

I was admitted to the hospital that morning and immediately started on fluids and one hundred milligrams of oral steroids. The steroids were in a blue bottle with *prednisolone* handwritten on it. The name might be slightly different, but I knew what was about to come with those tiny, bitter white pills.

"I'm already taking prednisone," I told him.

"Oh?" his eyebrows shot up. "What dosage?"

"Twenty."

"That's not enough to do you any good at all," he said.

"I know," I told him. "I was on a stronger dose, but the side effects were so bad that once my symptoms were under control, I asked for a lesser dosage."

"That's probably why you're here right now," he said, helping me walk from my chair and get into the little wooden bed. The sheets were blue. *Like the scrubs my doctors wear back home.* "Settle in, Danielle," he added. "You're going to be here a while."

I looked around at my new "home." The walls were bare, except for a few wires and unused nails, save one that held the IV bag

Dr. Stark's nurse had attached to my arm. Royal blue drapes donned the windows, and some sort of air tank sat next to the bed. The floors were covered in tan tile that had been ice-cold to my bare feet. The grout looked like it had seen many patients tread over it through the years, and a small line of diligent ants hugged the baseboards.

"Ryan." I grabbed his hand. "You'll stay with me, won't you? He *can* stay with me, can't he?" I all but begged Dr. Stark.

"Of course he can," Dr. Stark said, smiling. Then, after giving a few more orders to his nurse, he excused himself, promising to check in on me first thing in the morning.

My dad went back to the hotel to update the rest of the team on my condition while Ryan stayed behind with me. I felt terrible making him leave the comforts of the nicest hotel in Kampala, but I couldn't bear the thought of being alone.

———————————

Over the next three days, my fever continued to rise and my health continued to decline. The lack of nutrition, the dehydration, and the pain in my abdomen led to hourly dry heaves. I was still unable to keep anything down, so Dr. Stark switched me to eighty milligrams of steroids intravenously, which amplified the side effects tremendously. My heart raced so fast that I'd wake up in the middle of the night and think I was having a heart attack.

"Is this your normal heart rate?" Dr. Stark asked when he read my vitals, which the nurse had taken earlier in the day.

"It has been since she's been on the steroids," Ryan told him. "Why?"

He shook his head. "A normal resting heart rate is between sixty and one hundred. Yours is one hundred twenty." He shook his head. "You really shouldn't be here."

Ryan and I exchanged worried glances. I wondered if, like me, he was trying to figure out whether Dr. Stark meant that I shouldn't be in Uganda, or I shouldn't even be alive.

"Honestly, Dr. Stark," Ryan began, "if either of us had any idea that Danielle's condition was *this* serious or had the potential to get this bad, we *never* would have come on this trip."

"Never," I confirmed, shaking my head. "We even checked with my doctor before we left, and he said I could go."

Dr. Stark smiled sympathetically. "Well, he probably shouldn't have. Just sitting on a plane for hours can be extremely taxing on your system, especially if you are on the verge of a flare." He looked back down at my chart. "And I'm guessing you had some vaccinations before you left?"

"Yes." I nodded. "A lot of them."

"Were any of them 'live'?" he asked.

Ryan and I looked at each other. "I think two or three of them might have been," Ryan said.

"Well, that probably didn't help either," Dr. Stark replied. "Live vaccines can overstimulate the immune system, and your system is already overstimulated. That, combined with the stress of the trip, the cabin pressure, the different time zones . . . honestly, it would have been more unusual if this *hadn't* happened."

I spent the next few days lying in bed, kicking myself for being so naive. *What made me think I could handle a trip like this? I never should have come.* Even worse, because of me, Ryan was missing out on his trip of a lifetime as well. Instead of helping the other guys with the building projects they had planned and playing with the kids in the camps, he was stuck here in this dingy little hospital with me. I clutched his hand as he napped in the chair next to my bed and smiled. Despite everything I was dealing with, I couldn't help but marvel at what an amazing and sacrificial man my husband was. He never complained about anything. He just focused on caring for me. Every morning, he trekked across town on foot to get me juice, bottled water, and boxes of Ceres Nectar, which was my only source of calories. And every night he would climb into my bed, read to me from the little Bible we had brought, and pray.

After one particularly difficult night, Ryan read Psalm 91 to me. "I feel like this is what we're supposed to pray," he said, straining to read the tiny print in the poorly lit room. I felt comfort and hope as I listened to him read about how the Lord, our place of safety, will rescue those who call on him in trouble. How we don't need to "dread the disease that stalks in darkness" because the Lord will answer us in our trouble.

Ryan and I spent whatever lucid time I had reading through that psalm over and over and praying for God to turn this disease around in its tracks. When Ryan slept, I would slip on my earbuds and listen to one of my favorite worship songs, "When the Tears Fall." I clung to the words "When pain surrounds, I'll call You healer" and listened to the song on repeat.

I tried to believe those words. To let them comfort me. But it was easier said than done, lying in this unfamiliar country and in such uncertainty. I had grown up in the church, but until now, most of my prayers had been for small, more trivial things—a passing grade on a test, a good parking spot, a beautiful sunny day for my wedding. My faith had never really been tested before, and to be honest, I wasn't sure I was ready for it.

When Sunday morning rolled around, Ryan and I sat in the silence of the two-room hospital while most of the staff were off for the weekend or attending church in the city center. With what little strength I had left, I prayed that we would be given some sign of hope.

Then, off in the distance, I heard the most beautiful, worshipful singing. It sounded like the music I knew from church back home. The words were even in English. My eyes grew wide as I looked at Ryan.

"Do you hear that?"

He squinted his eyes, listening in earnest, then shook his head. "No."

"Okay," I sat up a little in my bed, "be really quiet and listen."

I held my breath as Ryan again concentrated on hearing the music. I knew the steroids sometimes caused me to hallucinate, and I wanted to make sure it wasn't happening again.

A slow grin spread across his face and he nodded. I grabbed his hand and tears streamed down my face as I listened to those pure voices singing a song of praise. Just as I was starting to feel alone and forgotten, a glimmer of hope wafted in with those voices floating through the air.

Moments after the singing ceased, Dr. Stark appeared in the doorway. He'd told us he didn't make rounds on the weekends, so I was surprised to see him and hoped his unscheduled arrival didn't mean bad news.

"I've just come from church," he said. "I felt God impress upon me that I was supposed to come and check on you. And pray for you."

Wow. I was stunned. We had never discussed our faith with Dr. Stark, so until that moment, I didn't even know that he believed in God.

"Were you attending the church nearby?" I asked. "We just heard them finish singing."

His face bore a quizzical look. "My church is ten kilometers away. What singing did you hear?"

I explained about the song I'd just heard, and he shook his head as if what I was saying was impossible. "I've never heard anyone worship nearby in the ten years I've been working here. The community that surrounds this hospital is not known for being one of faith."

I looked at Ryan for reassurance. *I did hear it, didn't I? I wasn't hallucinating?* Ryan smiled at me and nodded.

"Well then," the doctor said, "it seems God has you in Uganda for a special reason. Do you mind if I pray for you?"

"No, please, we'd love that," I said, wrapping Ryan's hands in both of mine.

As Dr. Stark prayed, I realized I had never had a Western-trained doctor do anything like that during any hospital or office visit. In my experience, faith and medicine were not intertwined. That morning restored a glimmer of hope in me. Someone greater than everything that was happening was with me, reminding me that he is good, even in times of desperation and hopelessness. *Maybe I* am *going to be okay.*

Another few days passed without my symptoms improving. In the eight days since I'd been in Uganda, I had lost fifteen pounds, and I still wasn't able to keep down food or most liquids. I was feeling particularly stir-crazy when Dr. Stark entered my room holding my test results and wearing a look of defeat.

"I'm afraid your hemoglobin levels are continuing to drop, which means your anemia is getting even worse." Then, his voice heavy with concern, he said, "There's nothing more I can do. Danielle, if you don't act quickly, your condition could be fatal. You need to return to the States for a blood transfusion and to access better medications, and you need to do it as soon as humanly possible."

I stared blankly at Ryan, the fear rising in my chest. I knew I was ill, but . . .

"You're saying I could die?" My voice was barely above a whisper.

Dr. Stark nodded solemnly. My stomach clenched—this time from panic. We needed to get home as quickly as possible.

The next day, Ryan and I said our goodbyes to the group and went back to the Entebbe airport to make our way home. I felt worse than I'd ever felt in my life. I had worked so hard to come here, hoping I'd have an opportunity to serve, to make some small difference in the lives of people who desperately needed help. Now I was leaving, and poor Ryan had missed out as well. I felt like I was letting everyone down. And I still couldn't wrap my head around Dr. Stark's dire warning. He said I needed to get home immediately. But home was still forty-eight long, hard travel hours away. *What if we don't make it in time? What if my body can't handle the trip?*

While Ryan and I had been making travel arrangements, his dad, Dwight, had been busy calling to get me an appointment with one of the best GI doctors in San Francisco. That doctor was booked for months, but somehow my father-in-law was able to pull a few strings and get me an appointment the day after we landed. So the plan was to get me home, let me sleep a bit to catch up from jet lag, and then see the doctor the following day.

As our plane lifted off, my stomach dropping in concert with the cabin pressure, I grasped Ryan's hand tightly and prayed. *God, please let me make it home safely.*

As Uganda slowly disappeared in the window, all our hopes were now pinned on this new doctor. *Please, God, let this doctor have the answers we're looking for.*

5

My appointment was scheduled for 9:00 a.m., and I hadn't slept well. Between the jet lag and the faintness from the loss of blood and lack of food, I couldn't even make it to our bedroom when we got home. I collapsed on the couch and spent the night there instead. Ryan helped me as I dragged myself to the car, and then he drove us to the appointment.

"Ryan, I don't think I'm going to make it," I said looking for a bench to rest on outside the medical center. People hurriedly walked by, and I felt myself grow jealous. It had been all I could do to walk from the car to the front door before needing to sit down. I was just thankful to be out of the wheelchairs that had pushed me through all the airports on our treacherous journey home.

When we finally got to the doctor's office, the room was already filled with patients, even at that early hour. I was astounded to see that most of them were young women who looked to be around my age.

"Danielle Walker," a pleasant-looking nurse called out. Ryan nodded and stood to lend an arm so I could follow behind the nurse. I assumed she was leading us into an exam room, but instead, she ushered us into a large office. "The doctor will be with you momentarily," she said, turning on her heel and heading back out front.

I glanced down at my hands folded in my lap. They were deathly pale, the bones in my wrist were protruding, and my fingers looked abnormally bony. I knew I'd dropped a lot of weight in the past ten days, but when I looked down at my body, I was stunned. My clothes, which fit perfectly two weeks ago, now hung off me, and I could clearly see my rib cage bulging beneath my skin.

How did I get this sick so quickly?

Just then, the door opened and an older gentleman in his early sixties with white hair and glasses walked in reading what I assumed was my file.

"Danielle? I'm Dr. Benedict." He looked up from the file and abruptly stopped, his eyes widening and his once-welcoming smile vanishing, replaced by a look of alarm. "We need to get you straight to the hospital."

"Why?" Ryan asked, mirroring the doctor's concern. "What's wrong?"

"We need to get some blood and nutrients in her as quickly as we can." He slipped around the back of his desk, picked up the phone, and directed the person on the other end of the line to bring blood-testing equipment to his office.

He's going to test me right here?

Within seconds, a different nurse appeared with a needle, tubes, and a small cup of apple juice.

"Here you go," she said kindly, offering me the juice. "Drink up so you don't pass out."

The nurse poked my right arm, drew blood—the dark red fluid

was a stark and shocking contrast to my translucent skin—and then left the room.

"What exactly do you know about your disease, Danielle?" Dr. Benedict asked.

"Not much," I admitted. "I know I have ulcerative colitis, and that it can cause anemia."

"That's right," he said. "And based on your appearance, I'm guessing you are severely anemic. I'm also guessing that you're either coming off of or are in the middle of a major flare-up. Is that right?"

I glanced at Ryan. Dr. Stark had used the term *flare-up* to describe what was happening in Uganda, but at the time, I was too weak to ask him what that meant. Sensing I was overwhelmed, Ryan stepped in and gave Dr. Benedict a quick rundown of the past two weeks. Nothing Ryan said seemed to take him by surprise.

"The doctor in Uganda called it an autoimmune disease," I broke in. "What does that mean?"

"Yes," Dr. Benedict explained, "ulcerative colitis *is* an autoimmune disease. What that basically means is that your immune system is mistakenly attacking an otherwise healthy organ—in your case," he said, nodding in the direction of my stomach, "your colon. Normally, your immune system guards your body against bad bacteria, viruses, and infections, and when it encounters them, it attacks and gets rid of them. Your immune system should be able to tell the difference between your own healthy cells and foreign cells. But when you have an autoimmune disease, your system *can't* tell the difference, and when stressed, it releases proteins called auto-antibodies that attack the healthy cells. That's what a flare-up is—your immune system is literally attacking you from the inside. About half of people with UC have mild symptoms," he continued, "but from what I'm seeing, your case looks to be pretty severe."

Ryan squeezed my hand.

"Some autoimmune diseases target only one organ," he continued.

"Type 1 diabetes, for example, attacks the pancreas; psoriasis, the skin; ulcerative colitis, the large intestine; Crohn's, the small intestines. Other diseases, like systemic lupus erythematosus, affect the whole body."

Oh my gosh. I couldn't even imagine how horrible it must be for those poor people.

"There are over eighty types of autoimmune diseases," he added, "and as many as fifty million people in the US alone suffer from them, hundreds of millions around the world."

At least I wasn't alone.

"But I'm only twenty-three," I said, as though that somehow negated everything he was saying.

He smiled sympathetically. "UC can happen at any age, but it's becoming more and more common to see patients develop it between the ages of fifteen and thirty. Truth be told, we see a lot of it in young twentysomethings like yourself." I thought back to the women in his waiting room. "Mostly type A personalities, people who deal with a lot of stress."

Okay, that *did* sound like me.

"The gastrointestinal tract is very sensitive to emotion," he explained. "Anger, anxiety, stress —all of these feelings can trigger symptoms in the gut."

"So are you saying that stress triggered all of this?" I asked.

"Not necessarily," he responded. "The truth is, we really don't know what causes autoimmune diseases. It could be hereditary or environmental factors, or a combination of the two. We do know that more women are affected than men, and that certain things like stress, viruses, bacterial infections—even antibiotics—can trigger autoimmune diseases."

My mind flashed back to a few months before our wedding when I was fighting that stomach bug and the doctor prescribed antibiotics. *Is that what caused this? Or was it the antibiotics coupled with the stress of the wedding?*

I ran my theory past Dr. Benedict.

"It's really impossible to say," he admitted. "You may have been carrying this gene for years and it was just waiting for the perfect storm to strike."

I wanted to cry, in part from exhaustion and in part because it felt so good to finally have someone explain what was happening to me. We continued to talk for a few more minutes until the nurse returned with my test results.

"Yep," Dr. Benedict confirmed. "You definitely need a blood transfusion. You are, as I suspected, severely anemic. The normal range for hemoglobin, which is a protein in red blood cells that carries oxygen throughout the body, is twelve to fifteen in women. You're at a six. If you drop any lower . . ." His words hung in the air. He never came right out and said it, but his meaning was clear. If I didn't get a transfusion immediately, I could die.

Once again, I was admitted to the hospital. They settled me into a massive room that was bright, white, and full of windows overlooking the San Francisco skyline. I thought back to my Kampala hospital experience. *What a stark contrast.* This bed moved and could rest at an angle. And there was a TV in the corner of the room with nurses coming and going all the time. The click of the IV machine in my room was so much noisier than the bag, dripping because of gravity, that had been hanging on a nail on the wall in Kampala. Somehow the simplicity of that room under Dr. Stark's care had felt more comforting.

They started the blood transfusion right away.

"Just don't look at the bag," one of the nurses told me as she hung a bag full of blood on a metal pole that connected straight to my arm via an IV. Of course, I looked. How could I not? It was so weird to see blood going in instead of out for a change.

Next up was the iron infusion. It stung and burned and throbbed like crazy.

"This really doesn't feel any better," I admitted to Ryan, who now looked almost as pale as I was.

They checked my levels again after the transfusion and saw that I still wasn't in the normal range, so they gave me a second bag of blood. Within twenty-four hours, I felt like a new person.

Though my UC symptoms weren't gone, I felt alive again. I had an appetite, and my energy level increased dramatically. I was still nowhere near my old self, but compared to where I was when I checked into the hospital, I was feeling worlds better. Two days later, Dr. Benedict released me, but not before prescribing more steroids and anti-inflammatory medications. He strongly advised me to stay off my feet for a few weeks until my symptoms abated and I could keep solid foods down and my weight up.

I took medical leave from my job, and over the next two months, my schedule consisted mostly of me sleeping on the couch and, if I was feeling up to it, taking a trip to the grocery store with my mom. One day I felt so good I decided to go to Trader Joe's by myself. I leaned heavily on the shopping cart to make it through the store, but by the time I got to the checkout line, I was so wiped out, I collapsed. I managed to catch myself before I caused too much damage, but it frightened me.

At my next appointment with Dr. Benedict, I told him what had happened, and he added some nutrients to my medical regime.

"I want you to get more potassium and iron in your system," he said. "Also try taking some omega-3 fish oil. It will help with the inflammation."

"Okay," I agreed. He was the first doctor to "prescribe" anything other than medications, which made me curious. "Is there anything else I can do on my own that will help?" I asked. "Change my diet or anything?"

He shook his head. "No. Changing your diet isn't going to heal you." I slumped down in my chair. It was the same thing Dr. Beale had said. "But," he continued, "for now at least, you may want to go off all things refined and white. No white flour, white sugar, or white pasta. They've been stripped of all their nutrients, and since your body desperately needs all the nutrients it can get, it will help if you eat foods that supply those nutrients, along with the vitamins I give you."

Wait. That's the exact opposite advice Dr. Beale gave me. "I thought you said changing my diet wouldn't change anything."

"It won't help your disease," he said. "That's what the medications are for. You just need more vitamins and minerals in your system after losing so much during the last flare-up, and whole wheat breads and pastas are loaded with them. Just try it for a few weeks, until you get your strength back up."

I couldn't quite make sense of what he was telling me. If it didn't matter what I ate, why had two different GI specialists specifically instructed me to eat totally different things? Dr. Stark had also said that the way food is grown and prepared can affect the body. Dr. Benedict just prescribed fish oil and potassium supplements— but weren't those two nutrients I could get by eating actual fish or bananas? Given that my particular disease involved the colon, where food is digested . . . weren't they *all* making the case that food *does* in fact play a role?

———————

By the end of 2008, I was mostly recovered and had been able to wean myself off the steroids. Per Dr. Benedict's recommendation, Ryan and I had started eating whole wheat everything—flour, bread, pasta, pizza, the works. It was pretty easy. I just swapped our frozen DiGiorno pizzas for their whole wheat version, our boxes of white pasta for the deeper-brown whole wheat pastas. When I baked, I used the fibrous whole wheat flour instead of the bleached all-purpose flour hiding out in my pantry.

My weight was back up, and my energy level had returned almost completely to normal. Now that I seemed to have the UC under control, I turned my attention back to the plans Ryan and I had made before the UC threw a wrench into everything—starting a family.

We had been trying for almost a year, and while I hadn't been in perfect health and it was probably best for my body not to carry a baby, I kept a close watch every month. When I finally missed my regular cycle, my stomach grew giddy with anticipation. I didn't tell Ryan because I wanted it to be a surprise. When the two little lines on the pregnancy test confirmed my suspicions, I was ecstatic! So was Ryan. Even my body began to feel wonderful again. The UC symptoms disappeared, and for the first time in over two years, I felt . . . normal.

Everything seemed to be going well, but I still headed into my ob-gyn's office for my first ultrasound armed with some questions. For example, I hadn't yet experienced some of the early signs of pregnancy that I had read about online, like morning sickness or the first telltale sign touted on all the pregnancy websites—enlarged and tender breasts. By my calculations, I was about ten weeks along, so I wondered if it might have just been too early.

As Dr. Veerman moved the ultrasound wand around, her face lit up. "Looks like two!"

Twins? Ryan and I each had twins in our families, but I always thought it skipped a generation. I was so excited that I barely registered the shift in my doctor's face from enthusiasm to concern and the subtle but swift turn of the ultrasound monitor away from my view.

"Let's see what's going on here," she said, studying the screen and moving the wand again to get a clearer picture. "You *do* have two yolk sacs. . . ." She paused for a second. "Something doesn't look right, though. See that flurry of white, snow-like specks there?" She shifted the monitor back my way and pointed to the screen. "That concerns me, but I do detect a faint heartbeat."

My breathing stopped. *This doesn't sound good.*

"But it's a little too soon to know definitively." She turned her full attention to me. "We're going to need to monitor you a little more closely. I'd like to have your blood tested every few days to monitor your placental hormone levels. That should provide us with some answers."

"My ulcerative colitis . . . ," I began. "Do you think that's causing—"

"No," she said, putting my mind to rest. "The medication you're on is a category B, which means it's safe for pregnancies. Let's not rush to conclusions. We'll just do some tests and see. But if you experience any cramping or bleeding, call me immediately, okay?"

I waited for the results and tried to go on with life. Then the call came.

"Danielle, I'm afraid your hCG numbers are even higher than I expected. I'd like to do another ultrasound, tomorrow if possible."

My eyes pricked with tears. The next day, Ryan sat holding my hand as Dr. Veerman once again ran the ultrasound wand over my stomach.

"Danielle, I'm afraid the babies have stopped growing," she said, a sorrowful tone in her voice. "And I'm not picking up any heartbeats. I believe you've experienced a molar pregnancy." She explained that not only had I lost the babies, but I would need to be monitored to ensure no tumor developed in my uterus.

Ryan and I drove home in silence, and I crawled into bed, fully expecting never to come out. The weeks following were the darkest moments I had ever experienced. I couldn't eat. I couldn't sleep. I couldn't be around anyone who had young children or was pregnant or watch anything on television that depicted the same.

My ob-gyn continued to monitor me through weekly blood tests to make sure my hormone levels were dropping to ensure a tumor wasn't forming. Thankfully, they fell at a healthy rate, which meant we could start thinking about pregnancy again in six months rather than twelve. I did my best to carry on while continuing to grieve, and I looked toward that six-month mark when we could try again to grow our family. But as my hormones began to return to normal levels, I started to get those all-too-familiar cramps. The emotional and physical stress was too much. I was heading toward another flare-up.

The problem was, the "cure"—steroids—was almost as bad as the disease. And I didn't want to go back down that road.

"Isn't there something else?" I asked Dr. Benedict at my next appointment. *"Anything?"*

He thought for a moment. "There's a relatively new drug for UC on the market. It's called Remicade. It's getting a good response, especially from patients who don't handle steroids well."

I leaned forward, feeling hopeful. *If he can keep me off steroids, I'm all in!*

"It's an immunosuppressant that's administered intravenously. You might compare it, in a sense, to chemo, but for autoimmune diseases." He explained that I'd have to go to an oncology clinic every six to eight weeks for a four- to five-hour session.

"Like chemo, it can shut down your immune system so that it doesn't act up. But—" he gave me a sad smile—"one of the potential side effects is that you'd be susceptible to every cold and flu. We'd also have to test you for tuberculosis before starting the treatments because it could be fatal if you caught it while on the medication."

"What about pregnancy?" I asked. "Could I carry a baby to term successfully?"

He shook his head and winced a little. "I'm afraid there isn't much research on that yet. The drug's too new."

That frightened me. "Could I discontinue and then restart it?" I asked, figuring that I could just go off it during pregnancies and then continue after giving birth.

He shook his head again. "No. If you went off it, your body

would build antibodies to it, rendering it ineffective if you tried to go back on."

"I don't think I'm quite ready for that yet," I admitted.

"Danielle," he said solemnly, "your condition is extremely volatile. You aren't going to be able to predict when a flare-up will happen. You may go six months to a year before the next one. But given how severe your case is, it could also be a month. The flare-up could last a few days, a few weeks, or even a few months, and the recovery could take just as long. We need to do something. I know you don't like the steroids, but it's either that or the Remicade."

"Thank you, Dr. Benedict," Ryan said. "We'll think about it."

That night, Ryan and I were despondent.

"So those are our choices?" I sighed. "Debilitating steroids or life-long 'chemo' treatments?"

"Don't worry, babe," Ryan assured me. "I'm sure there's another option. We just haven't found it yet."

"I know," I smiled weakly. "I just hope we find it soon."

———————

"I can't believe I didn't think of this sooner," my friend Jeanine chirped into the phone, "but I know a woman named Susan whose teenage daughter has the same thing you have—and she is in complete remission! Maybe you should get together with her and ask how she did it."

"Are you kidding me? Of *course* I want to meet her!" I'd never met another girl who had my disease, let alone someone who had found a way to manage it.

The following week, Ryan and I met with the mom at a local Starbucks. As we sat outside at a table, soaking up the sun's rays, she began telling us her daughter's story.

"No medication," she claimed. "We did it all by supplements and vitamins."

The more she talked, the more hopeful I became. I could do this! I could take those supplements too. If they worked for her daughter, they should work for me!

"I went ahead and made up a list," she said, pulling a long hand-written list out of her purse. I looked it over. I had never heard of most of the items on it. But she swore by them all. So after our meeting, Ryan and I headed directly to the nearest health-food store and bought every single one.

"I really hope these work!" I said, looking at the receipt and seeing how much we'd paid.

"Well, if they do, it will be more than worth it," Ryan confirmed.

That night, after I took my regular prescription, I went down her list, item by item, and gulped down the written amounts for each supplement.

I hope these are the right amounts for me. I knew there were different dosages for different people, but I had no idea how to figure out what they were, so I just took what she told me to and hoped for the best.

"So," Ryan asked one evening, "are they working?"

I had been taking everything on the list for several weeks now, and honestly . . . I had no idea whether they were working or not. In some ways I felt better, but the cramping seemed to be worse. The problem was, I didn't know which supplements might be helping and which ones might be hurting, so after a few months, I just stopped taking them.

"I don't think these are doing the same thing for me that they did for her," I reluctantly told Ryan as I packed hundreds of dollars' worth of half-empty bottles into a box and stuck them in the back of the closet.

"Maybe one size doesn't fit all," Ryan suggested, rubbing my back. "It was worth a try."

I appreciated his optimism, but to be honest, after failing to find success with MiraLAX, the refined white foods, the steroids, the whole wheat, and the small fortune in supplements I was now boxing up, I was tired of trying.

––––––––––––

"So how are you getting along?" God bless Jeanine. She knew I had been struggling, so she made a point of stopping by the office one afternoon to check on me.

"Not great," I admitted.

"Here," she said, pulling a book out of her bag and placing it on my desk. Multicolored vegetables that looked to have been drawn in the eighties surrounded the book's title, *Breaking the Vicious Cycle: Intestinal Health through Diet*. "I heard about this through somebody who has similar struggles. I don't know what it is, but maybe it will work for you, too." She smiled and shrugged.

"Thanks," I said thumbing through the pages. "That was very sweet of you." After Jeanine left, I spent some time skimming the table of contents and introduction. The book seemed to focus on something called the Specific Carbohydrate Diet and the impact certain foods and chemicals had on the digestive system. *I don't want to read about the science*, I thought, closing the book and slipping it into my bag. *I just want someone to tell me what to do to make it better.*

I appreciated the gesture. I knew Jeanine's intentions were good. And I knew she had experienced relief from multiple sclerosis through dietary and lifestyle changes. But I'd had my fill of the "try this" and "try that" approach. I was just worn out. So that night when I got home, I put it up on our bookshelf, along with all the other books I owned but had never read.

A few days later I was cooking pasta for dinner. As I dropped the noodles into the boiling water, I glanced at the box. It was regular pasta, not whole wheat.

I had felt a tiny bit better when I stopped eating the refined and white foods. Maybe I should go back to eating whole wheat.

The thought stayed with me after dinner. *Maybe I can find something online that talks about other foods that might help.*

All the doctors said food couldn't cure my disease.

What if they're wrong? I quickly shook the idea from my head. Doctors spend years studying the body. They know how it works. Who was I to question them? Then again, even my specialists didn't seem to agree on what worked and what didn't—high fiber, no fiber, white, wheat. *Maybe Ryan's right. Maybe there is another option.*

I opened up my laptop and googled "food and ulcerative colitis," but nothing came up. *Okay,* I thought, *how about "food and autoimmune diseases"?* A few sites popped up, but most of them simply explained what an autoimmune disease was. I decided to check some medical chat forums, after making sure Ryan was fully engrossed in his law school studies in the next room. Since my last Google search had almost resulted in me making my own funeral arrangements, I had promised him I wouldn't try to self-diagnose anymore. *I'm just doing a little constructive research,* I thought as I smiled to myself.

I found one forum on colitis and Crohn's and read some of the posts, which might have been interesting had I not been looking for something more practical. But then I noticed a small tab at the top of one of the pages linking to a subforum on food, so I clicked it.

Several people on that page mentioned going gluten-free. I had seen a few gluten-free items in the grocery store, but I wasn't entirely sure what gluten was. A few others mentioned they were doing the Specific Carbohydrate Diet (SCD), and it was helping.

Specific Carbohydrate Diet. Where have I heard that before? I racked my brain, trying to remember. Then I noticed the bookcase. *Of course! That book Jeanine gave me.* I picked it back up and scanned through a bit of it. The author, Elaine Gottschall, said that she created the diet for her daughter, who suffered from ulcerative colitis, and her daughter went into complete remission.

Complete remission! Now *that* got my attention. I glanced at what the diet entailed. That got my attention too. It looked pretty strict. No grains. No lactose. No processed or canned foods. No chocolate.

What else is there? I looked at the gluten-free option. That seemed more doable. I still wasn't sure what gluten was or why it made a difference, and frankly, I didn't care. As long as I could still eat the foods I loved, what difference did it make if they were made with white flour, wheat flour, or gluten-free flour?

The next morning, I went to the store and grabbed anything labeled "gluten free"—doughnuts, waffles, pizza, pasta, and bread. And over the next several weeks, my symptoms seemed to calm down a bit.

Finally, I thought. I had found the solution I'd been looking for! I went through my kitchen cabinets, refrigerator, and freezer and pulled out all the whole wheat foods I could find (as whole wheat and gluten seemed to be pretty much synonymous) and gave them to friends, family members, and coworkers. *No point in letting it all go to waste.*

After I finished making my deliveries, I collapsed on the sofa and breathed a deep sigh of relief. At last I was sure I was on the path toward remission. After spending more than a year puzzling over conflicting doctors' orders and suffering the debilitating side effects of multiple medications, I was finally taking control of my own health.

And to think, all I had to do was stop eating gluten. Maybe food did have something to do with my illness after all.

PART 2

Eat Well

6

"I'm going to introduce you to Becky and her husband, Ben," my friend Karis said, taking a sip of coffee. "They live right down the block from you guys. I think you'd totally hit it off."

"I don't know, Karis," I hedged. Shortly after returning from Uganda, Ryan and I had moved into a new neighborhood, but my flare-ups had kept us from being as social as we normally would have been.

"I think you'd really like them," she insisted. "Ben is a pastor at our church. They've got a little girl who is two, but they struggled with a lot of infertility issues before having her."

That struck a chord. Though we were trying our best to move forward, Ryan and I were both still reeling from the loss of our twins. And because Karis and I worked in the same office, she was one of the first to know about it, and she understood the grief I was still processing.

"Maybe it would be good for you guys to get to know each other," Karis suggested.

She had a point. "Okay," I agreed.

"Great!" she said. "I'll give her a call and tell her to expect you."

It turned out that Becky and Ben lived just three doors down from us. And Karis was right—I liked Becky instantly. She was warm and friendly, and she had the most adorable little girl I had ever seen. While Ryan and Ben wandered off to talk about craft coffee, Becky, two-year-old Maddie, and I played on the floor in the living room. Maddie was equal parts sweet and sassy, and just being there with her—given Becky and Ben's history—gave me hope that I might one day have a little girl of my own.

"We need to have you two over for dinner," Becky said as soon as Ben and Ryan came back into the room.

"That would be great," Ryan said, beaming. Clearly he and Ben had hit it off as well. I nodded my consent, but in the back of my mind, I was a little nervous. *How do I bring up the gluten-free thing?*

Before I could even mention it, Becky chirped in with "Do you guys have any food allergies?"

My eyebrows shot up in surprise. I had never had anyone ask me that before—even before the UC. Still, what if she didn't know what gluten-free was? What if it was too much of a hassle for her to make something I could actually eat and they never invited us back again? I bit my lower lip and glanced at Ryan, who nodded encouragingly. *Well, since she has been gracious enough to ask . . .* "Actually," I said apologetically, "I just started eating gluten-free." I held my breath.

Becky smiled brightly. "No problem."

My jaw dropped. *She knows what gluten-free is!* I exhaled into a relieved chuckle and said, "Thank you!"

"Of course!" she said, smiling, before turning her attention back to Maddie.

A few days later, we walked hand in hand back to their house for dinner. Ben, Ryan, and I spent the first part of the evening playing on the floor with Maddie while Becky was in the kitchen finishing up dinner. At one point, I poked my head in, offering to help. Whatever she was making smelled amazing.

"That looks wonderful," I told her, peeking over her shoulder into a serving dish brimming with roasted chicken and potatoes.

"Thank you," she said. "And don't worry, it's all gluten-free."

I was so appreciative that she had cared enough about my needs to accommodate me, even though I never really expected her to. "Thank you so much for going out of your way like this," I told her.

She just waved me off. "Oh, it wasn't a problem at all. I'm on a special diet myself because I have ulcerative colitis."

She has UC? Becky and I had spent the better part of an afternoon earlier that week talking all about Maddie, their move to the area, and Ben's role in starting a new church, and she never once mentioned having UC. Then again, I never mentioned that I had it either. It's not something you just drop into casual conversation. I stared blankly at Becky, my mouth hanging open in stunned silence. She looked . . . healthy. *She's healthy* and *she has had a baby.*

"Are you all right?" Becky asked.

It was only then that I realized I was crying.

"I was diagnosed with ulcerative colitis two years ago," I managed to choke out. "It's been so miserable, and then this spring Ryan and I lost . . ." My voice cracked, and Becky reached over and put her hand on my arm.

"I know." Becky smiled kindly.

"You look fantastic," I offered, smiling through tears.

"I've been in remission for two years."

Two years! When I finally got my voice back, I asked her about her experience with drugs, doctors, and diet.

"Yeah, they all told me the same thing," she said. "That food has no bearing on the disease. But I've had no flare-ups, and I'm sure it's because of the food I've been eating. Or not eating."

"What diet are you on?" I asked.

"The Specific Carbohydrate Diet, or SCD, as the insiders call it." She winked.

There's that diet again! That was it. Becky had sold me. Even though the people on the chat boards were very positive about the plan, I didn't know any of them. I didn't know their circumstances. But to see another woman my age—with a family—who credited the diet for putting her in remission? How could I not at least try it? Eating gluten-free seemed to help a little, but I was still having symptoms, so maybe I needed to take it one step further.

As soon as Ryan and I got home, I marched over to the bookshelf and pulled down the book Jeanine had given me.

"Talk about an answer to prayer, huh?" Ryan said, settling in on the sofa next to me. "I mean, what are the odds we'd move into a house three doors down from someone with the same condition you have?" He was right. In fact, I almost felt guilty. Ever since we'd returned from Uganda, I had been so frustrated with God. First that disastrous trip, then the loss of the babies. And none of my doctors seemed to agree on anything or have any viable long-term solutions to help me manage this ridiculous disease. All this time I'd been praying for healing, and when it didn't miraculously happen, I started to wonder if God was even listening. Now I knew. Not only had he been listening, but little by little, he'd been dropping answers to my questions right in my lap—first Dr. Stark's revelations about gut health, then this book from Jeanine, and now Becky. Maybe God had always been listening and I just wasn't hearing it. Or maybe it was that he'd answered in ways I hadn't expected. But now I suddenly felt more hopeful than I had since this whole nightmare started. *I can do this*, I thought, opening the book to chapter 1. *I can figure this out. I will figure this out!*

Still not interested in the science behind the diet or how the colon works, I quickly jumped to the back of the book, where the author had included lists of what to eat and what to avoid. There were even a handful of recipes. *Yes!*

I scanned the allowed, or "legal," list: vegetables, unprocessed meats, eggs, natural hard cheeses without lactose, homemade yogurt, fruit and all-fruit juices, nuts, unrefined oils, unflavored gelatin, weak tea and coffee, mustard, vinegar, and honey. That seemed doable.

Then I looked more closely at the unacceptable "illegal" foods: refined sugars, all grains, all canned foods, some legumes, starchy vegetables, complex carbohydrates, canned and processed meats, milk, cream, soft cheeses, baking powder, balsamic vinegar, candy, chocolate, carob.

No chocolate. No bread. And no baguettes with cheese. No more of my new go-to gluten-free pasta with a jar of store-bought sauce. No more heaping bowls of oatmeal in the morning and ice cream or frozen yogurt at night.

Basically, SCD was grain-free, lactose-free, and free of complex carbohydrates and anything refined or canned. I got the refined piece, thanks to Dr. Stark. The canned stuff, I assumed, was off-limits for much the same reason—all the preservatives required to keep otherwise perishable foods shelf stable and edible for months, if not *years*, longer than nature intended. I scanned a little further down the page and found a list of grains on the list of banned foods— wheat, barley, rye, millet, sorghum, rice, oats, and even corn. *Okay, wheat, barley, and rye, I get. It's the gluten. But what's wrong with the other ones? And how is corn a grain?* I made a mental note to do some additional research into the effect of grains on the body.

The good news was that the author said some foods, like certain dairy or beans, could be eaten, but not until they had been either fermented or soaked and then slow cooked.

Ugh. Fermented milk? I stuck out my tongue. *Why bother?* But then the image of Becky, thriving and playing with her two-year-old daughter, flashed through my mind. *It's okay*, I assured myself. *You can do this.*

I flipped back to the recipe section and looked for one to get started on. I found a basic chicken soup recipe that didn't look too difficult. I read the ingredients: chicken, water, carrots, onions, celery, parsley, and a little salt.

Seems easy enough.

I continued scanning the recipes. I could have homemade Jell-O made from gelatin and 100 percent grape or unfiltered apple juice, not from concentrate. I could also have applesauce, but it had to be homemade and really cooked down well, especially while symptoms were present. I read further to find that raw fruits and vegetables were hard on the digestive system, but once cooked, their nutrients and sugars were easily transported through the bloodstream. And the author suggested I introduce daily yogurt into my regimen, but again, I would have to make it myself.

The only yogurts I knew of were in the grocery aisle, but those were full of sugar and hadn't been fermented long enough to reduce the lactose or increase the beneficial bacteria much. How long was yogurt supposed to ferment? I wondered. A paragraph later, I got my answer—twenty-four hours. *Twenty-four hours? Holy cow. Better get crackin' on that!*

I grabbed my laptop, went to Amazon, and typed in "yogurt maker." I'd never been a huge yogurt fan, but I figured I could get used to it. As I read the recipe—take milk, add a yogurt starter, then let it ferment for sixteen to twenty-four hours—I thought back to what Dr. Stark had told me about how powerful good bacteria is for the gut, and in a small way, I started to feel empowered. I was finally taking control of my health, and I was grateful for the role Dr. Stark played in that.

The next morning, I went to the store and bought all the ingredients I needed to get started. The first week, I could eat a little bit of yogurt, some soup, eggs, and gelatin during the day. Then for dinner, I could have a plain hamburger patty or a piece of salmon.

When I phoned Becky to tell her I'd gotten the yogurt maker and was starting the diet, she said, "That's great! Hold on, though. I have some chicken soup already made that I can bring you." Minutes later she was standing at my door. As she gave me a big glass container, she said, "You're going to be eating this three times a day for a week, so this should be enough for you not to run out."

I had envisioned a colorful, delicious-smelling soup with big juicy chunks of chicken swimming in a clear yellow broth, dotted with tiny sliced carrots and crisp celery rounds—like the kind my mom would make when my siblings and I were sick. But when I looked in Becky's container, the entire top was covered in a thick layer of fat and the cold liquid base of the soup seemed to jiggle like the jellylike goo in the movie *Flubber* when I shook the container. "Thank you," I said as pleasantly as I could, hoping against all hope she hadn't registered my initial shock.

"Don't let the fat or gelatin bother you," she said. *So much for that.* "It helps heal your gut and allows you to absorb nutrients better, but it's also going to sustain you through the days since you won't be eating that much."

"Okay," I said, wondering how in the world I was going to swallow all that fat.

"You'll want to ease into your first week," Becky explained. "Just stick to the soup, cooked vegetables, and cooked fruits. In fact, I know it will sound odd," she continued, "but for breakfast, you'll want to eat the soup. The broth will help to heal your gut, so you want to eat it as often as you can stomach it." She spent some time explaining the diet further and encouraging me as I started it. She also warned me that I might actually regress before getting better. That part scared me.

The next morning, I pulled the container out of the fridge and stared at that thick layer of fat. *It may be healthy, but it sure isn't appetizing*, I thought as I poured some of it into a pot and heated it. Thankfully the gelatinous broth turned to liquid as soon as it hit the heat. But when I tried to eat it, I just couldn't get it down—the slimy texture of the fat was too much for me to handle.

Then I decided to make my own soup. I already had the ingredients. I tweaked the recipe a bit by taking the skin off the chicken and skimming off a bit of the fat, even though the book said I was supposed to leave some. *It might not be as filling*, I reasoned, *but neither is skipping breakfast entirely because it's inedible.*

The experiment with the yogurt went better—at least for me.

"Try this," I said placing a small bowl of homemade yogurt in front of Ryan.

His face scrunched up as he looked at it. "What is it?"

"Yogurt. It's easy to make, so I'm going to stop buying the regular stuff."

He took one bite and almost spit it out. "I love you, Danielle," he said, "but this is terrible. It's so sour!"

He wasn't wrong. It *was* pretty sour. But that's because I couldn't add sweeteners—they increase the pathogenic (bad) bacteria in the gut. *Maybe if I add some fruit to it*, I thought. As Ryan tucked into a bowl of cereal, I looked over at the fruit bowl on the counter. *Hmm . . .* I could have bananas. The book said so. I grabbed a spoon and a small bowl, broke the banana into little pieces, mashed it up, mixed it into the yogurt Ryan had set aside, and took a bite. *That's not bad*, I thought, taking a second bite. *Not bad at all, in fact. Maybe this is doable.*

I was grateful for this bit of hope because eliminating all grains, as the SCD required, was a big challenge in itself. By now I had figured out what gluten is. It's basically a protein-based binding agent found in wheat and some other grains like barley that makes things like bread and pasta dough stretchy, and once baked, helps them retain their shape. It has little inherent nutritional value, and its "gluey" nature makes it difficult to break down, which can wreak havoc on the digestive system.

I knew bread, bagels, pasta, and pizza dough were obvious culprits, but when I'd begun reading lists of ingredients on food labels, I discovered that gluten also shows up in many foods I never would have expected—things like hot dogs and sausages, soy sauce, salad dressings, soups and soup mixes, gravy, frozen french fries, and pre-seasoned frozen vegetables. I even found it listed in some of my cosmetic and hair products!

And I had to be careful because not all ingredient labels included the word *gluten*. I also had to keep an eye out for anything that *contains* gluten. Wheat, for example, shows up in imitation seafood, frozen turkey patties, marinara sauce, and virtually every boxed breakfast cereal in our pantry, not to mention three of my favorite *C*s—cookies, crackers, and croutons. Even seemingly healthy foods like oatmeal, granola, and muesli could be off-limits if they were cross-contaminated or included flour as a binder.

Within a week of starting to follow the SCD, I did start to notice a slight change in my body. Though my symptoms didn't completely disappear, I didn't need to go to the bathroom nearly as much, and the bleeding and cramping slowed down significantly.

After the intro week, I was able to start adding in the other items on the allowed list. That helped, but everything tasted so bland and drab. I tried making simple pancakes that contained almond butter, zucchini, and banana, but they tasted like cardboard and the texture seemed, well . . . weird. And since Ryan wasn't following the diet, I was essentially making two meals every night. In the interest of saving time, I did my best to keep them the same—if we had burgers, for instance, I'd give him a bun and eat mine without. Then I started making food to freeze, so I could just pull it out and reheat it, but it was really time-consuming. Honestly, it wasn't easy cooking something I couldn't eat either; I felt taunted with every stir as the aromas wafted into the air. Instead of looking forward to meals, by the end of the third week, I was starting to dread them.

It was gut-wrenching, in more ways than one. Food had always been something to enjoy and celebrate over with friends and family. This diet might be helping alleviate my symptoms, but it gave me nothing to look forward to, nothing to revel in. I just missed eating. *How am I supposed to go out with friends or family if this is all I can eat?* I wondered. *How does Becky do it?*

A few weeks later, my efforts resulted in the runny cauliflower disaster when Ryan and I went to our friends' Friendsgiving. I wanted to contribute something I could eat, so I made mashed cauliflower "potatoes," which turned out more like soup. As everyone piled their plates high with all the traditional goodies of the holiday, loaded with sugar, gluten, starchy vegetables, and processed foods, I sat at the end of the table with a plate of plain turkey (I had to pass on the gravy) and runny cauliflower mashed "potatoes." I felt so left out watching everybody else feast on things I didn't dare touch.

I looked down at my plate. *In the US alone, about 50 million people suffer from autoimmune diseases and another 32 million have food allergies, and this is the best we can do? This terrible food that sucks the joy out of us?* I couldn't stand the thought that I would be reduced to eating nothing but broiled chicken, runny cauliflower, and banana yogurt if I wanted to be healthy.

Why not create my own recipes? I mused. *I figured out the banana hack. I'm sure I could come up with other ways to make this stuff taste better.*

There was only one problem. Though I liked to cook, I had never actually made up my own recipes for anything before. Still, I reasoned, it couldn't be any worse than this.

———————————

The next day, armed with my "legal" and "illegal" food lists, I headed off to the grocery store to seek out the ingredients I needed. *I hope this works*, I thought as I watched the checkout total go higher than I was used to spending. I headed home to start experimenting. Muffins would be my first venture.

I excitedly pulled out one of my banana muffin recipes and looked it over. I could substitute a lot of the ingredients to make them work for me. Where the recipe called for a cup of bleached all-purpose wheat flour, I substituted a cup of almond flour. I couldn't have sugar, but I was allowed honey, so I swapped that in. And instead of cow's milk, I used an equal amount of almond milk.

I made every substitution at a 1:1 ratio. It quickly became clear that would not work. Those overly dense, greasy, gritty-tasting muffins went to Ryan's office and to our parents with a caveat of "These aren't great, but I'm working on something new!"

I went back to the drawing board and tried the muffins again, tweaking a little here, substituting a little there. In place of butter, I tried coconut oil. I kept the honey, added three eggs, vanilla extract, three bananas, baking soda, salt, and cinnamon. Then I began adding almond flour in small increments until . . .

"Perfect!" The muffins were warm, and the taste was so reminiscent of the banana bread I'd grown up with that I ate two of them. I had done it! I had proved that I could eat healthy and not deprive my taste buds of pleasure. And if banana muffins could taste delicious, what else could?

I turned my sights to peanut butter cookies. I had eaten some of the premade gluten-free ones from the grocery store, but they just weren't as good as homemade. They were too crumbly and dry. I grabbed one of my mom's recipes and started substituting "legal" ingredients. I bought organic peanut butter made from peanuts and salt only (no sugar added) but kept the softened butter, baking soda, eggs, salt, and cinnamon, and then substituted honey for sugar and almond flour in place of regular flour. The consistency of the dough didn't look quite right, but I pressed the tines of the fork into the batter to make the traditional grid pattern nevertheless. Act as if, right? And to my surprise, they baked up great!

"This is pretty good," Ryan said, a note of surprise in his voice, as he munched on one of the cookies.

"Thanks!"

"You've been working hard on these recipes," he said, taking another bite. "Maybe you should start a blog. Share them with your family."

A blog? I did love writing in college. And it would save me from having to retell my story every time we got together with family or friends. *Still . . . me write a blog?*

I flashed back to how I'd felt when I found one of the only food blogs that dealt with restrictive diets and how much hope it had brought me when I needed to know I wasn't alone. I was proud of the recipes I had created. And I really wanted people like me to be able to eat good food again.

Maybe if I started a blog, I could actually help people. I giggled at the thought. *Who's going to read my blog? Nobody knows me except my family. And they'll probably only read it to be nice. And anyway, who will trust my credibility as a cook or baker? I'm not trained.*

As if reading my thoughts, Ryan gave me a hug. "Just share your story and what you're learning. If nobody reads it, that's okay. At a minimum, it will be a good creative outlet for you. But I bet more people will find you online than you can imagine. And I bet they're out there just waiting for someone to offer them hope."

"Okay," I responded with a nervous smile. "Let's do it!"

That night, Ryan helped me set up a basic WordPress site, but I struggled to come up with a name for it. One of the blogs I liked reading was Comfy Belly, so I tried creating alternatives to that, like Healthy Tummy, but they all sounded too cheesy.

Maybe it should be something about grains, I thought. Whenever family and friends would ask, "What can't you eat?" I would tell them, "I have to take out all grains."

"What about Against All Grain?" I asked Ryan. "You know, since I can't eat any grains and I always feel like I'm swimming upstream and going against the grain?"

"Yeah." He smiled brightly. "I like it."

I decided to post a mini frittata recipe I'd recently created. I wrote up a brief intro, which said, "I was running out of options for break-fast items that were quick before work, so I came up with these mini egg frittatas. I make a large batch of them every couple of weeks and freeze them individually so I can pop one in the microwave." I typed in the recipe, uploaded a grainy and very yellow-toned photo that I took on my smartphone, and then clicked on Publish.

One evening after deciding that I'd finally landed on the per-fect formula for a basil-thyme vinaigrette, I drizzled it over a fresh spinach salad. My excitement about creating a zesty dressing slowly turned to aggravation as I took photo after photo, trying to get one that would look good on my blog.

"You know," I told Ryan, "I wish I had a digital camera. My phone is okay, but the pictures don't really do the food justice. And they all look yellowish. I'm planning to photograph a few Thanksgiving recipes in the next few weeks; and I really want the photos to match how good the food tastes so people may be more willing to try them."

That Saturday morning, Ryan woke me up early and asked me to walk downstairs with him. Right away I noticed the crackling flames in our fireplace, but then he guided me toward a two-foot-tall artificial Christmas tree. Underneath was a box wrapped in fes-tive paper.

He handed me the gift but then said, "Wait!"

Now he was the one fiddling with his camera. Once the video was rolling, he said, "Okay! Open it."

I carefully unwrapped the paper from a box containing a little Canon Rebel. "You remembered! Thank you! Now I have a camera, a fire in the fireplace, *and* a Christmas tree!"

As I hugged Ryan, I wondered, *What can I possibly give him that would top this?*

7

I had my answer by the time we put up our real Christmas tree three weeks later—a positive pregnancy test! I felt as if I floated through the holiday season. I love Christmas anyway, and we had something extra special to celebrate this year.

A few weeks later, I smiled and patted my ever-growing baby bump as I sat in Dr. Veerman's exam room for a regular prenatal checkup. *I just know 2010 is going to be a great year!* I was continuing to follow the Specific Carbohydrate Diet, but the baby was healthy and growing, and for the first time in months, I was completely symptom-free. It was almost as if overnight, my UC had waved and said good-bye. I could tolerate food, I wasn't using the bathroom any more than a normal person, and I had zero bleeding. Even better, I actually had energy! In fact, I felt better than I had in over two years.

"How are you feeling?" Dr. Veerman asked.

"Great," I said, beaming. "Better than great. I feel fantastic!"

She smiled. "A lot of times pregnancy masks or alleviates the disease's symptoms."

"Really?"

"Yeah, when a woman is pregnant, her immune system essentially shuts down because if it didn't, her body would instinctively want to reject the fetus as a 'foreign entity.' Some women even stay in remission well after giving birth."

That would be awesome, I thought. For now, however, I was just happy that both the baby and I were healthy.

Regardless, I still tried to stick to my diet. One morning, however, I went to make myself a batch of my favorite banana muffins. As soon as I opened the bag of almond flour, the smell made me sick to my stomach.

That's weird, I thought. Then something occurred to me. *Maybe I don't need to eat this way right now. I mean, I feel great. And if the pregnancy has put me into full remission . . .*

Before I knew it, I had reverted to eating whatever I wanted—pizza, bread, ice cream, french fries—everything I thought I'd sworn off for good.

If it was filled with off-limits stuff, I was all in. If a pizza commercial came on the television, I *had* to have pizza. There was a place up the road from us that had the best buttery-garlic crust and little round pepperoni slices that pooled with the delicious grease from the cheese. And they had the best ranch dressing in the world to dip your slices in. But I didn't just crave pizza. I also craved Chinese food. Deliveries of beef and broccoli in a salty brown sauce were frequent during those earlier months of pregnancy, along with crunchy spring rolls and a side order of pork pot stickers. And of course I also reveled in Mexican food with luscious piles of refried beans, reminiscent of those Sunday taco dinners in Colorado. And for breakfast? Special K with strawberries. I couldn't get enough milk and cereal.

Ryan indulged me most of the time, but he did make me commit to one thing. He made me "sleep" on my cravings for at least forty-eight hours. "If you're still dreaming about it in two days, we'll get it for you," he told me.

In my thirty-seventh week, I held Ryan to that deal. I had a craving for a certain fast-food burger that I hadn't eaten since college after watching *Super Size Me*, a documentary about a man who goes on a thirty-day fast-food binge to explore the consequences of such a lifestyle. But now, almost five months after the craving hit, I still wanted that burger! True to his word, Ryan drove me to a nearby restaurant and pulled into the drive-through line, where I promptly ordered everything I used to eat in college—a burger, some chicken nuggets, fries, and a chocolate shake to dip the fries in (obviously). I didn't even wait until we got home to dig in. I just had Ryan pull into a parking spot. The smell of the food permeated the car. My mouth was watering, and I swear that little life inside me started doing somersaults at the scents. Then I took that first precious bite and was totally and completely . . . disappointed.

"This tastes nothing like I remember," I confessed as I looked down at the flimsy and greasy patty sandwiched between a deflated-looking bun. "It's actually kind of disgusting."

"Well," Ryan pointed out, "you've gotten used to eating much healthier." He was right. I had grown accustomed to the rich tastes and textures of real, healthy food and didn't even realize it. We finished what we paid for, but I never craved anything from that place again.

On August 16, one week after Ryan passed the bar exam, I went into labor. I was so excited to finally meet that little face I had been dreaming about. To kiss the tiny feet that had been relentlessly kicking me in the ribs for the last two trimesters. To find out if those little eyes would be blue like Ryan's or brown like mine. To see those ten little fingers and ten little toes, and to hold that precious little bundle for the very first time. And to open up the door to the bedroom I had closed and refused to step foot in for the past year and a half after losing the twins.

Because a friend had told me you're not allowed to eat once you're admitted and in full labor, I ate one last panini on San Francisco sourdough, grilled with tomatoes, melted cheese, pesto, and prosciutto. Then we packed a bag and headed off to the hospital. I had come to loathe visiting the hospital, but this time, I could barely contain my excitement.

After thirty-six hours of labor and no progression, Dr. Veerman decided to perform a cesarean section. She explained that they were going to start an antibiotic through my IV while they prepped me. Exhausted, I took in every word. *Antibiotics* and a *C-section*. I flashed back to what Dr. Stark had said about cesarean babies being more susceptible to autoimmune diseases, as well as his comments on antibiotics.

"We need to act quickly," Dr. Veerman said. "The baby's heart rate is starting to show irregularities."

Despite my initial denial and frustration—and lots of tears—I opted to do whatever it took to get my baby here safely and quickly.

Our beautiful son Asher made his way into the world and into my arms on August 18 in the early morning hours. His name means "happy and blessed"—precisely how we felt after grieving through such a long season of loss and illness.

I left my job to be a stay-at-home mom, and as the months went by, I settled comfortably into this new life of feedings, changing poopy diapers, and focusing on Asher's every need. He kept me busy, distracted, and extremely happy. I spent Asher's nap times testing recipes again as I began eating more grain-free as a precaution. I also resumed writing on the blog that I had neglected during most of my pregnancy.

It's hard to explain the enormous relief that comes with not thinking about your illness every waking minute. I relished relief from my symptoms and freedom from the fears and worries that had plagued me for so long: *Will I end up in the hospital again? What can I eat? What should I eat? Should I schedule that trip, plan that date night, commit to that activity—or will I end up doubled over in pain, having to cancel at the last minute?* It was a year of blissful reprieve, and I soaked up every minute.

———————————

By April 2011, Asher was eight months old, and we were introducing more and more solid foods. I nursed him at night, but during the day I supplemented with milk I had pumped and frozen earlier.

Then I noticed I was starting to use the bathroom much more frequently. A few weeks later, I spotted blood, but I swallowed down my fear. *It's nothing serious. I'm just overly tired.*

"Let's take a nap, Asher," I said, picking him up and carrying him to the bedroom.

When I awoke, I rushed to the bathroom.

Okay, no problem. I'll just go back to the first week of the SCD and dive back in. That afternoon, I cooked up a batch of the chicken soup and pulled out the yogurt machine. With every bite, my mind pleaded with the food, *Please work, please.*

It didn't. The pain slammed into me like a semitruck, and all I could do was lie in bed and suffer. Within a matter of weeks, large dark circles had formed under my eyes, my cheekbones were protruding, and my body looked positively skeletal. When I picked up a brush and ran it through my hair, clumps of long, brown locks pulled right out. *What in the world?* I pulled the hair out of the brush and stared at it. It looked like a bird's nest, all dry and brittle. When I looked back into the mirror, I barely recognized myself.

Even worse, no matter how hard I tried, I just could not muster enough energy to take care of Asher. I used to love sitting up with him at night to nurse. It was our special time together—something only we could do. But now his cries would awaken me in the middle of the night, and all I could do was listen as Ryan comforted, fed, or changed him. I could deal with my dark circles, thinning hair, and skeletal frame. But to not be able to take care of my own son when he cried ... that hurt me far more than my worst UC symptoms ever could.

"Do you want to make an appointment with Dr. Benedict?" Ryan asked. "I know you don't want to do the steroids, but the soup and yogurt don't seem to be working and we have to try something."

I sighed heavily and agreed.

"Let's talk about getting you on Remicade," Dr. Benedict said.

We knew that was coming. But infusions every eight weeks and compromised immunity for the rest of my life? *I'll never be able to go to any of Asher's school functions or classroom parties without worrying about picking up a bug and likely taking longer to recover from it.* No. I couldn't live that way.

Ryan spoke up. "We'd like to wait thirty days. See if we can get this under control with some other, less invasive methods." He looked at me, confirming what we'd already agreed to. "Then if absolutely nothing else works, we'll try the Remicade."

"Okay," Dr. Benedict reluctantly agreed. "In the meantime, I'll make out another prescription for prednisone and increase your dose of the anti-inflammatory mesalamine."

I thought about the dreadful side effects I'd suffered before and hoped against all odds that this time things would be better.

They weren't. Almost immediately after starting the steroids, all the side effects returned—the sleeplessness, racing heartbeat, blurry vision, puffy moon face—the whole nine yards. Worse was the zero tolerance and patience for my sweet baby boy.

My mom came and helped out as much as she could while Ryan was at work. One day, while we were talking about my frustration with the treatment, a small smile slid across her face.

"Seems like getting pregnant with Asher stopped the disease in its tracks," she said. "Maybe you should just be pregnant all the time."

"Ha!" I laughed. "How many grandkids would you like—five, ten?"

I had to admit, pregnancy was definitely preferable to Remicade. But ultimately neither was an ideal long-term solution. Still, we had thirty days to make one last-ditch effort.

Jeanine had told me about an integrative wellness center in Southern California that specializes in treating autoimmune diseases with supplements and alternative forms of homeopathic healing. We decided it was worth trying, so we packed up Asher and headed south.

For the next two weeks, I was given daily vitamin C infusions and a low dose of naltrexone cream, which was supposed to increase endorphins and modulate the immune system so it wouldn't attack itself further. But that was only the beginning. I also tried acupuncture, infrared light therapy, L-glutamine supplements, and even nicotine patches, which studies had shown could suppress the immune system, decrease the inflammation of ulcerative colitis, and boost production of the mucus in the colon that acts as a protective barrier. I've never been a smoker, so all those patches did was make me nauseous. I also tried a sludgy-textured drink called bentonite clay, which was supposed to provide minerals, repair my colon, and detoxify my body, as well as a handful of other supplements, many of which had been on the list my friend had given me after we got back from Uganda.

After two weeks, we returned home, our savings drained to zero. I was in even worse shape than before.

"Do you think *anything* they tried helped?" Ryan asked.

I shook my head. "I don't know. Maybe we tried too many things at once. How are you supposed to know what's working and what isn't?" One of the things I liked about the Specific Carbohydrate Diet was that it started by taking everything down to zero—just eating the soup, then slowly adding other things in one at a time. At least that way you could monitor your symptoms and see what moved the needle. From what I learned from Dr. Stark and Dr. Benedict, my immune system was already in overdrive. Throwing everything but the kitchen sink at it all at once probably made it worse. In fact, I was *sure* it had.

Nothing seemed to be working. And the prednisone was suffocating me, giving me hallucinations, and making me feel as though my heart was going to just cut out, so I quit taking it. Cold turkey. My doctor had given me a strong warning against doing that, but I was so desperate I didn't even consider the danger. Unfortunately, stopping it just made everything worse. I became so incapacitated that I could no longer spend *any* time with Asher. Most days when Ryan would bring him into my room, I had to turn him away. My little boy would inch his way around my bed, holding on with both hands and sidestep until he reached me, then he'd look at me with his pleading blue eyes to pick him up. All I could do was look at him and cry. Then Asher would start crying because I couldn't play with him, and Ryan would have to remove him from the room, while he stretched his little arms out begging me to take him. It was torture.

I knew supplements could help. They certainly worked for Susan's daughter. And so many people on those chat boards said they worked for them, too. *Maybe supplements work differently for different people? Or maybe I just need different dosages?* Ryan and I both knew people who had found relief from chronic illnesses by using infrared light therapy and acupuncture. And the Specific Carbohydrate Diet was doing wonders for Becky. Even *I* had experienced some success with it.

Of course, Becky's UC symptoms got worse during pregnancy while mine disappeared completely. Clearly this was not a one-size-fits-all disease. Why would the treatment be any different? Just because these things hadn't worked for me didn't mean they didn't work at all. Plus, I reminded myself, I wasn't just trying to manage normal symptoms, I was trying to combat a major flare-up.

"I'm starting to wonder if the answer is a combination of food, supplements, and . . . I don't know . . . something else," I told Ryan. "Maybe my body is just too far gone this time to accept the homeopathic treatments and we need to get it back to ground zero with medications so we can try the alternative methods again."

Whatever the solution was, one thing was certain—we were running out of time. Within the past month, I had lost nearly twenty-five pounds and was suffering from severe arthritis-type pain. It felt as though somebody were chipping at my bones with a hammer. I could barely even walk.

"We have to take you to the hospital, Danielle," Ryan finally said. "We said we would give it one more chance by going down to Southern California, but we don't have a choice now. This is really bad." His face looked genuinely concerned. It was the same look he had when we were in Uganda.

I nodded slowly. I felt so defeated. I knew that if I went back to the hospital, I would be forced back on the steroids, but this wasn't just about me anymore. I had to find a way to get better—for Asher.

While I lay on a gurney in one of the ER rooms waiting for a doctor to see me, Ryan talked with Dr. Benedict over the phone.

"She needs to go back on medication immediately," Dr. Benedict told him.

"No," Ryan shot back. "We're not doing the steroids. Isn't there *anything* else besides Remicade? Any alternative medications? What about the Specific Carbohydrate Diet? We know someone who has been in remission for over three years now because of the way she's been eating."

"I told you already that food won't cure her," Dr. Benedict said flatly. "It won't alleviate her symptoms. It won't put her in remission. Her disease is one of the most severe cases I've ever seen."

"Well, she can't do the steroids anymore," Ryan countered. "It just makes her worse. She literally can't survive on them."

"So you're saying you refuse to do the prednisone?" Dr. Benedict asked.

Ryan looked at me, and I nodded. "Yes."

"Mr. Walker, you're going to kill your wife if you won't allow her to go on the necessary medications."

"But what about—" Ryan began.

"I'm telling you," Dr. Benedict said with an edge to his voice that I could hear two feet away, "there *is* nothing else. If you're not going to follow my instructions, then I'm afraid there's nothing more I can do to help you."

Ryan looked down at his phone and then over at me.

"What did he say?" I asked.

Ryan sighed and raked his fingers through his hair. "I think he just fired us."

8

"Now what do we do?" I asked Ryan.

He shrugged. "We get another physician." He smiled gently and took my hand. "For now, let's see what this ER doctor can come up with."

When I told the doctor about my symptoms—in particular, the intense joint and bone pain—not only did the hospital admit me, they quarantined me and sent for an infectious disease specialist.

"Our insurance company is going to love us," Ryan whispered to me, lightening the mood as we waited for the results from my blood tests.

"Mrs. Walker?" the doctor said, pulling back the exam room curtain. "Your tests don't show any infectious diseases."

That was a plus.

"We believe your inflammation has spread beyond your digestive system into other parts of your body."

"Can you do something to stop that?" Ryan asked.

Looking at me, the doctor said, "We should get you on ster—"

"No," I said firmly, cutting him off. "No steroids." Both Ryan and the doctor looked stunned. The doctor, I got. They all seemed equally taken aback by my refusal to take the steroids. Ryan . . . I think he was just shocked to see me take such a determined stand. Truthfully, so was I. Up until now, I'd pretty much done whatever the doctors ordered. After all, they were the specialists. But were they experts when it came to me and my body? I was genuinely starting to wonder.

"Okay," he said reluctantly. Instead he put me on an IV with fluids and a series of antibiotics to help control the inflammation and combat any potential infections. He ordered both a blood transfusion and an iron infusion to address the anemia and dehydration. He also put me on a liquid diet to give my colon a break and help with the inflammation.

Within a day or two, I began to feel my energy and appetite restored. In fact, I felt so good that I wasn't even panicked over having lost one of the best gastroenterologists in California. *Who needs a GI doctor anyway?* I mused. *Especially if all he's going to do is prescribe what he's always prescribed, regardless of my specific needs.* But now what?

Becky's face floated back through my mind. She'd been in remission for years now. Why couldn't I do that? There was no doubt in my mind. Food had to be the answer.

As soon as we got home, I pulled out *Breaking the Vicious Cycle* and started thumbing through it again. *This has to work.* I thought about all the online testimonies I'd read about those who followed SCD or the Gut and Psychology Syndrome (GAPS) diet, which was modeled after SCD. Both focused on eliminating bad bacteria and healing the gut by replacing difficult-to-digest foods with nutrient-dense and gut-flora-building ones. The remissions I read about were a direct result of the food these people were eating and avoiding—not the medications. That couldn't be a coincidence.

I whipped up another batch of chicken soup and more almond flour banana muffins. The SCD had improved my symptoms before I got pregnant. Maybe I just hadn't stuck with it long enough.

The following day my sister-in-law, Jeanne, called to check up on me. "Listen," she said, "I've been seeing a naturopath, Dr. Walters, and she's amazing." I knew Jeanne had been struggling with some digestive and hormonal imbalances and had been trying alternative treatments for that. "She's got me on some supplements and foods specific to my particular issues that have helped my symptoms all but disappear. Maybe you should give her a try."

Food specific to her particular issues? That piqued my interest. "What's her number?"

Two days later, Ryan and I walked into Dr. Walters's office. I looked around at the simple décor. There was no front desk or anyone waiting to sign us in.

"Danielle?" A petite woman stepped into the main room and greeted me. I expected her to be much older, but she appeared to be in her thirties. Her eyes sparkled.

I think I'm going to like her.

She listened closely, nodded, and took notes as I told her about my symptoms and everything I'd tried. Then she put down her pen and gave me the sweetest smile. "Let's get you some help, okay?"

That one sentence brought me more peace and comfort than I'd felt from medical professionals in years. I almost cried right then— and she hadn't even started!

"The body can react to foods in many different ways. Adverse food reactions can lead to distressing symptoms and chronic health conditions. So first, we need to figure out what is right for you. Food isn't a blanket, one-size-fits-all formula to healing and health. Certainly, some things apply to everybody, like the need for vitamins and minerals and the elimination of foods like dairy and grains to help decrease inflammation, but this is a bit different. You noticed improvement with SCD, but there may be some foods you were still eating that your body doesn't respond well to, especially when it's in crisis mode. We need to cater to *your* body so we can see optimal health, yes?"

What she said made sense. I thought back to all those supplements I'd taken based on what Susan's teenage daughter took. How different might the outcome have been had I been able to customize them to fit my own needs? And when I tried SCD, I didn't veer from the protocol at all, fearing it might not work if I did. But I wasn't really paying attention to my symptoms or watching how those foods affected me.

"We're going to do some testing," Dr. Walters told me. "Comprehensive stool analysis to look for inflammation, bacteria, yeast, and parasites. A comprehensive nutritional panel to see what vitamins and minerals you are deficient in. And a blood test to look for antibodies to foods and environmental allergies so we can see how you respond."

"I'm sorry," I interrupted. "Antibodies?"

"Sorry." She smiled before explaining further. "The blood test measures antibodies—blood proteins produced in response to and to counteract specific antigens—to eighty-seven commonly consumed foods. Antigens are toxins or other foreign substances that induce an immune response in the body, especially the production of antibodies. The test is not 100 percent accurate or a final fix, but it's a good place to start."

"Okay," I agreed. "Is there anything I should do in the meantime?"

"For now, you can follow the Specific Carbohydrate Diet," she said. "We'll look at the results and go from there, okay?"

As I waited on the test results, I stuck strictly to SCD, still seeing only marginal improvement. I couldn't understand why it had worked so well for Becky but wasn't giving me the same results.

The following week, Ryan and I went back to Dr. Walters's office.

"Okay," she said, flipping open a file with my name on it. "It looks like you have some minor sensitivities to cinnamon, cilantro, and egg whites. You also have some more serious sensitivities."

"You can tell that just from a blood test?" I asked.

She nodded and passed a small white card across the desk to me. "These are the foods you need to avoid right now," she explained, "because you have sensitivities to all of them."

I looked down at the card. It was filled. In addition to the three foods she'd already mentioned, I saw a long list: Asparagus. Baker's yeast. Beef. Brewer's yeast. Buttermilk. Casein. Cottage cheese. Cow's milk. Gluten. Goat's milk. Kale. Kiwi. Lamb. Millet. Mozzarella cheese. Onion. Oregano. Parmesan cheese. Parsley. Pea, Green. Peach. Pineapple. Potato. Raspberry. Safflower oil. Sage.

I looked up at Dr. Walters in disbelief. Then she reached across the desk and flipped the card over. Spelt. Swiss cheese. Watermelon. Whey. White mushroom. Wild rice. Yogurt. Zucchini.

"Wow," I said. "That's . . . a lot."

"Yes, but that's good." She smiled. "Now we have a direction to go in. And some of these may have shown up because you had eaten them in close proximity to the testing."

I glanced at Ryan and smiled hopefully.

"Now that we know your food sensitivities," she continued, "we're going to do what we call an elimination diet. That basically means we're going to take you off everything except a few basic items we know you aren't allergic to. We'll start by eliminating all the items on this card, and then add back in the items that are likely to be benign, like the seasonings and herbs. We'll slowly add the more inflammatory foods in one at a time and see how your body reacts. By isolating the different foods, we'll get a clearer picture of which ones are actually causing the problems."

My eyes widened. That is *exactly* what I had been thinking at the wellness center. *Maybe I understand all this better than I thought!*

As Dr. Walters listed all the items she wanted me to eliminate, I just about passed out. I wouldn't be able to eat eggs, nightshades (i.e., tomatoes, eggplant, peppers, white potatoes), nuts, seeds, grains, legumes, dairy (including fermented or lactose-free), refined sugars, or anything raw.

Wow, I thought. *What's left?*

"Just for the time being," she said, reading my thoughts.

I looked back at the list and my eyes zeroed in on yogurt. "I've been making this SCD yogurt, and it's fermented. Is that why SCD wasn't completely working for me?" I asked. "Because I was eating yogurt, which I have a sensitivity to?"

She smiled and nodded. "It's possible, yes. Cow's milk and casein are also on your list, which are both in that yogurt you've been making. Fermented foods are very good, but right now, because of where you are health-wise, you need to take a break from it all. You might be able to add *some* dairy back in—especially goat's milk dairy because it has a different protein structure—once your body has healed. But for right now, I need you to be very strict."

I continued to scan the list. "I also make these almond flour muffins. And I've been getting a lot of my calories right now through seeds and nuts. I put almond butter in my smoothies, and I've been eating a lot of salads."

She shook her head apologetically. "Don't eat any salads. And you'll have to stop eating the muffins for now as well. Almonds can be difficult on the digestive system and cause inflammation if you're not able to digest them properly. Your colon needs as big a break as possible for the time being."

"But what else am I going to eat?"

"Cooked vegetables and meat, for starters. And I'd like you to keep a journal of your symptoms. Take note of what you eat and how you feel afterward, good or bad. That will give us a road map moving forward."

As much as I could see the logic in what she was saying, I had to admit, this elimination diet seemed *much* more restrictive than the SCD—and that one was brutal!

"I know it seems difficult, Danielle, but remember, it isn't forever," she assured me. "Trust me; you're going to see a difference very quickly."

In addition to my food lists, she sent me home with a myriad of gut-healing and anti-inflammatory supplements: probiotics to replenish the beneficial gut bacteria I'd lost with the last round of antibiotics and as a supplement since I could no longer eat yogurt and other fermented foods; herbs and supplements for gut soothing and healing (aloe, marshmallow root, slippery elm, licorice root powder, L-glutamine); supplements for inflammation (fish oil, turmeric); and vitamins and minerals I had grown deficient in (vitamin B, iron, potassium). I took a deep breath as I looked at the many bottles. Each represented an additional expense on top of our out-of-pocket fees for the tests and appointments with Dr. Walters, which insurance wouldn't cover.

I recognized a lot of the supplements from Susan's list. Maybe this time, with the help of a practitioner, they would work for me. "Record your experiences when you add each supplement back into your diet and bring it on your follow-up visit so I can give you better guidance."

"I really liked those muffins," I lamented to Ryan in the car. "And no nuts?"

"Just give it a try, Danielle," he said.

That night I made myself a piece of salmon, simply roasted with only salt and no extra oil, and a cup of chicken bone broth. For breakfast the next morning, I warmed up another cup of broth and had some applesauce that I'd made in the slow cooker.

The first two days were harsh. All I wanted was to get back the strength I needed to at least pick up Asher from his crib. I had barely any energy and felt nauseated most of the day. But by the third day, something changed. As I scanned the tally marks in the top right-hand corner of my food journal, I couldn't believe my eyes. When I first went to see Dr. Walters, I was still vomiting frequently and going to the bathroom upward of twenty-five times each day. But within just forty-eight hours of eating this way, I was down to six to eight times a day—a 75 percent improvement in just two days! (In case you were wondering, this is the way those of us with an inflammatory bowel disease measure our symptoms.)

So food really did make a difference! It was all I could do not to burst into tears. *If food can bring about this drastic of a change so quickly*, I wondered, *what would happen if I went all in?*

I'd dabbled with diets before, but I'd never really gotten serious about the way I ate. Even when I was doing the SCD, whenever we went out to eat or were at someone else's house for dinner or a party, I would give myself permission to have a bite of this and a taste of that so I wouldn't offend anyone. But before, it was just Ryan and me I had to worry about. Now there was this little life who depended on his mother to be there for him. To provide for him. How could I do that if I couldn't stay well for more than a few months at a time? I'd already missed his first step. I wanted to be there when he started walking for real. I wanted to be there for his baseball games. I did not want him to grow up hearing me say, "Mommy can't make it to your school play today because I have to stay in bed."

It was time to trust that food really could be the solution and go all in. For Asher.

I worked with Dr. Walters for months to determine which foods were working well with my system and which ones weren't. Which supplements were causing me more distress and which ones were helping. Which dosages worked best for my body. It was brutal. We had cut out all the spices and herbs on my list, which in my mind meant no flavor. How could I make all my fall favorites without cinnamon? Or my Mexican dishes without cilantro?

About six months after I eliminated all the potentially inflammatory foods, I began reintroducing foods into my system. I did it very slowly in a nuanced way. First, egg yolks. When I reacted well to those, I tried egg whites, separately, a few days later. When that went well, I ate the yolks and the whites at the same time. It was official—my system could handle eggs. Next came almonds. Then walnuts, then cashews, then sesame seeds. One at a time, we added back everything on my list, with two main exceptions—grains and dairy.

"Those," Dr. Walters explained, "are going to be out for at least a couple of years, and maybe forever."

My shoulders slumped.

"I know," she said. "But grains and dairy are common triggers among people with UC, Crohn's, IBS . . . all the inflammatory bowel diseases. They are also problems for those who are trying to heal a leaky gut, which allows toxins and irritants to seep into tissues outside the intestines. You appear to have this condition as well. Grains and dairy are just too difficult to break down. And given the severity of your condition, it's not worth the risk."

It was disappointing, but honestly, given what I already knew about gluten and inflammation, I wasn't surprised. What *did* surprise me were some of the foods that caused my symptoms to increase, namely dairy, beans, onions, and garlic.

"You put onions and garlic in the SCD chicken soup, right?" Ryan asked when I told him.

"Yes. I was also putting soaked beans in soups and chili because SCD said I could. And I was eating that yogurt every morning. That's probably why my symptoms never completely went away." It all made sense. I had blinders on and couldn't see anything outside of the "legal" and "illegal" SCD guidelines in my periphery.

Becky and I may have had the same disease, but we had different food sensitivities. Once again, the one-size-fits-all approach wouldn't work.

So it was not just the food itself; it was what was in it, how it was digested, and how it was prepared. That made me think, *Maybe it wouldn't hurt to learn just a little of the science behind it*. I turned on my laptop and found the website related to the book *Breaking the Vicious Cycle*. I clicked on the tab "Science behind the Diet" and read this:

> The Specific Carbohydrate Diet™ is predicated on the
> understanding that Ulcerative Colitis, Crohn's Disease,
> Irritable Bowel Syndrome, and gluten therapy resistant
> Celiac are the consequence of an overgrowth and imbalance
> of intestinal microbial flora. By altering the nutrition we
> take in, we can affect the constitution of our intestinal flora,
> and bring it back into balance, healing our digestive tracts
> and restoring proper absorption.

I had to look up a few of those words in the dictionary, but thought, *That seems logical enough*. The article explained that more than four hundred bacterial species—some benign, others not—live in the intestinal tract. In a healthy gut, communities of microbes exist in a state of balance. *The microbiome. Just like Dr. Stark said*, I thought. When that balance is upset, the intestinal flora can proliferate rapidly, which can worsen the production of gas and acids, inhibit absorption of nutrients, trigger chronic diarrhea, and create additional mucus and other harmful by-products—all of which can further damage and ulcerate the intestinal surfaces. *So that's where the term* ulcerative colitis *comes from*, I thought. My mind flashed back to the crippling balloon-bursting bloating and pain during the MiraLAX— wheat bran incident.

> The Specific Carbohydrate Diet™ is based on the principle
> that specifically selected carbohydrates, requiring minimal
> digestive processes, are well absorbed and leave virtually
> none to be used for furthering microbial overgrowth in the
> intestine.

The web page went on to explain that as the microbes in the intestine decrease, gut health is restored so that cells throughout the body can be properly nourished. This includes those in the immune system, which is then able to fight against any microbial invasion.

I looked away from my monitor. It all sounded so . . . medical. And so obvious. Why were none of my doctors aware of this?

Now that I was officially down the rabbit hole, I decided to do a little more research, starting with what I knew I could eat—meat, vegetables, and eggs. I quickly learned that the *quality* of food we eat makes almost as big a difference as the *kind* of food we eat.

I thought back to when I was breastfeeding Asher. He was colicky and had really bad gas, baby acne, and eczema. At the time, I wondered if something I was eating might be causing it. Now I knew. Whatever my food had ingested, I ingested. And whatever I ingested, Asher ingested—a percentage, anyway. It was all connected.

"Do they make grain-free cows?" Ryan asked one night, only half-joking.

"Actually, they do!" I said, pulling up one of my new favorite websites.

"Here," I turned my screen so he could see it. "It says 100 percent grass-fed *and* finished beef is the healthiest kind of beef you can buy. This meat contains higher levels of omega-3 fatty acids and is also high in antioxidants, beta-carotene, vitamin D, and vitamin E."

"So the cows are basically organic then?" He leaned in to take a closer look.

"No," I said, scrolling down a little further. "See—right here it says even organic dairy cows can be fed organic soy, wheat, and corn. So . . . no pesticides, synthetic hormones, or antibiotics, but still not totally grain-free."

"Well, they certainly *look* happy." Ryan nodded at the image of the cows roaming freely in a bright green pasture.

I smiled. "Not only do these cows get to graze freely on pesticide-free grass and hay, but they also benefit from being outdoors all day absorbing sunshine and vitamin D. A lot of cows living in conventional dairy production farms barely even see the sun—or a pasture. They're stuck inside most of the day, crammed together in stalls eating chemical-laden, mass-produced feed out of a trough." The very thought of it made me want to cry.

"You've really done your research," he said, giving my shoulder a gentle squeeze.

"It's fascinating, really," I said, clicking on a hyperlink about the science behind pasture-raised and grass-fed poultry and cattle. "But basically, it all boils down to the fact that healthy animals produce healthy foods. It's the same thing with chickens and eggs. A lot of the mass-production farms use grain-based feeds and keep their chickens cooped up indoors all day without any room to roam free or spend time in the sun. Chickens are meant to be foragers and eat whatever they can peck from the ground—insects, greens, grubs." I shook my head in frustration.

"And everything in their system ends up in ours," Ryan said, finishing my thought.

"Yep." I released a heavy sigh. "And that's just meat. We also ingest all the chemical pesticides that are sprayed on crops." I turned to face him. "Did you know there are even genetically modified vegetables and fruits now? They insert a gene that makes vegetables more resistant to drought or chemical herbicides, or to make them grow faster and stronger."

"Just like God intended," Ryan said, chuckling before taking a sip of coffee.

"Actually, it's funny you mention that." I turned back to my laptop. "I keep coming across this thing called the Paleo diet. It's almost like a prehistoric way of eating, focusing on the foods bodies were originally intended to eat. Here," I said, pulling up another site. "It says that on this diet you can only eat fish; grass-fed, pasture-raised meats; fruits and vegetables; seeds and nuts; healthy oils and fats. You can't have any grains including corn, legumes including soy, dairy, refined sugars, refined or hydrogenated oils, or processed foods. Basically, it eliminates anything our prehistoric ancestors wouldn't have foraged or hunted."

"So you're just eating—" Ryan began.

"What God intended—" I continued, clicking back over to the site on grass-finished beef—"the way God intended it."

After almost three years of doctors, specialists, scans, tests, antibiotics, steroids, transfusions, and infusions, this was the first solution that actually made sense to me. God made our bodies to function well. And he gave us everything we need to keep them functioning that way. I'd tried the medical approach. Now, maybe, it was time to get back to basics. To try a more natural approach.

"Are you going to give this Paleo thing a try?" Ryan asked.

"I think I might. In some ways, it's similar to SCD—both cut back on carbohydrates and avoid all grains, refined sugars, and packaged or processed foods, and both focus on eating nutrient-dense whole foods, like meat, vegetables, and homemade bone broth. And it's already so close to what my food sensitivity test and Dr. Walters had me doing."

"So what's the difference?" he leaned back in to get a better look at the screen.

"Of the two, Paleo seems less restrictive, though it does cut dairy and legumes completely out. Of course, I can't have either of those anyway." I thought for a second. "I do like the gut-healing benefits of SCD—nothing raw while I'm symptomatic; fermented foods to rebuild my gut flora, that kind of thing."

I had pulled the SCD book off the bookshelf and picked it up. "Of course, some of the rules in the book are a little outdated. Canned and jarred products are both listed as 'illegal,' for example, but since this book came out, they've introduced a lot of healthy products into the market, so that takes the pressure off having to cook everything from scratch. That's a plus. And SCD doesn't focus as much on the quality of the food, whereas Paleo is all about nutrient density and buying the best quality proteins and produce you can find and afford. I like that."

"So . . . what's the answer?"

I thought about that for a minute. "Well, most of what I'm doing now with Dr. Walters seems to be leading down the Paleo path anyway, so I think I might try a combination of the two—but geared toward my specific needs."

Ryan nodded in approval. "That makes sense."

I sat back in my chair, Jeanine's book in my lap and a pasture of happy cows grazing on the screen in front of me. "Yeah." I smiled. "It does."

9

Grandma Marge's meat sauce . . . *Nope.*

Mom's shepherd's pie . . . *Nope.*

Nanny's beef stew . . . *Nope.*

Grandma Bonnie's sour meatballs . . . *Nope.*

One by one, I flipped through the recipe cards my family had given me at my bridal shower just a few short years before, looking for something—*anything*—I could still eat. One by one, they wafted gently to the floor. *I can't have any of these on this diet*, I lamented, then quickly caught myself. *No, Danielle, remember what Dr. Walters said.* I could picture her giving me a gentle but serious look as she told me, "This isn't a diet. This is for the rest of your life. Diets are only temporary. This is just the way you eat now. A lifestyle."

She was right. I had finally come to grips with the fact that this disease was not going away. It might go into remission for months—years even—but it would always be there. Contrary to what my doctors had been telling me, I was now convinced that the food I ate had the power to either alleviate or aggravate my gut issues. If I focused on eating the things that minimized the inflammation that exacerbated my condition, I could avoid the flare-ups that had dominated my life over the past few years. If I went back to eating the way I had before, I would eventually end up back in the hospital, unable to be the kind of mom I wanted to be for Asher—and any future children Ryan and I might have.

That didn't mean I didn't grieve the loss of all the comfort foods I'd grown up with and loved—Grandma Marge's tortellini; layered lasagna with cheese that stretched and pulled as you lifted a slice out of the tray; deli sandwiches loaded with meats, cheese, and mayonnaise on crusty baguettes; ice cream; frozen pizza; boxed Stove Top Stuffing at Thanksgiving; powdered sugar doughnuts at Halloween; french fries and burgers with buns when we went out to eat—those all needed to be things of the past.

I never knew you could mourn food. It was a strange feeling. Or maybe I was mourning the traditions that accompanied the food. We were still going to my grandparents' house nearly every month for the family feasts. And even though Grandma Marge always had a printed recipe from my blog neatly propped against the plexiglass window of a cookbook stand, the finished product lovingly prepared for me to eat, I hated that I couldn't eat all the other delicious food she set out on the buffet.

And what about the parties and gatherings I wanted to host? Would anyone want to come to my house for Thanksgiving if I couldn't even make or eat all the traditional foods people expect to enjoy on that holiday? And if they did come over for a meal or celebration to be kind, would they dread it or eat beforehand to be safe? Or come with the intention of running through In-N-Out for a Double-Double afterward?

This lifestyle change was necessary and would help me heal, but it would take a lot of getting used to. Ryan, Asher, and I continued to eat separate meals, for the most part. I would make a main dish we could all eat—such as salmon or roast chicken—but then I'd make something extra just for them, like rolls, rice, or fries. And I continued to buy all the traditional kids' snacks for Asher—cheese crackers, Cheerios, puffs. Of course, sometimes temptation would get the best of me and I would take a forkful off Ryan's plate and eat it or mindlessly nibble on scraps from Asher's high-chair tray while I cleaned up. After all, I reasoned, *One bite won't hurt, right?*

One night Ryan caught me doing it and shot me a "you know better than that" look.

"This is really hard," I mumbled, swallowing a leftover fry.

"I know. But how are you feeling?" Ryan said.

"Good," I admitted.

"And we know it's because of the food, right?"

I nodded reluctantly.

He paused. "Do you need me to go on this with you so you can stick to it?"

My heart leapt. "Yeah, that would actually be *really* helpful," I blurted out. Then the guilt hit. "But you don't *have* to eat this way . . ."

He just smiled, reached over, and took my hand. "I want you to be healthy. Asher needs a healthy mom. If it would help for all of us to eat the same things, then that's what we'll do."

I could feel the tears forming. *How did I ever get this lucky?*

"I'm just happy we won't have to eat that sour yogurt anymore," he added, laughing.

Amen to that. Of course, if both of us were going to be eating this way now, I definitely needed to find a few more options. Ryan's loving sacrifice was just the proverbial kick in the pants I needed. *I may have to eat differently from everyone else, but that doesn't mean I can't still have the kind of dishes I used to love.* I wanted to be the mom who makes chocolate chip cookies with her kids or bakes their birthday cake with them. But I wanted to eat that cake too. And dunk a still-warm cookie into a glass of milk at the counter with my kids. I knew I just needed to substitute grain-free, dairy-free ingredients in place of the things I couldn't eat anymore.

As I scraped the last remnants of french fries off Ryan's plate into the sink, I realized I needed to do one more thing—get rid of everything in our house that was not Paleo friendly. *Why flirt with temptation?* I thought, flipping on the disposal and watching those last few delectable wedges of deep-fried starch disappear down the drain. *Out of sight, out of mind.*

The next morning, I went through every cabinet and cupboard in our kitchen and bagged up every food item I was no longer allowed to have. As Asher played nearby, I pored over ingredient lists and, when in doubt, checked them against the SCD book and Paleo sites I had bookmarked.

It was harder than I expected. I had purged our pantry when I switched from whole wheat to gluten-free, but a lot of boxes and packets had crept back in, and this new lifestyle was even more limited. As more and more groceries disappeared from the cabinet and refrigerator shelves, my mind reeled over all the money I was wasting. *There has to be well over a hundred dollars' worth of food here*, I thought, looking over at the "gotta go" heap. Piled high on my table were containers of all-purpose flour, soy sauce, canola oil, cornstarch, condensed milk, peanut butter, bread crumbs, French's fried onions (for Mom's shepherd's pie and Thanksgiving green bean casserole), white sugar, and lasagna noodles.

The single-ingredient items like cornstarch, cornmeal, flour, and sugar were pretty self-explanatory and easy to weed out. The processed foods were trickier; it took a lot of research and reading to determine what could stay. Anything with grains, gluten, white sugar, peanuts, corn, or any corn product like high-fructose corn syrup was out.

I flipped over the box of cocoa mix with mini marshmallows that I'd bought on our last visit to Tahoe to visit Ryan's parents. Surely cocoa couldn't be that offensive? Though I knew chocolate was off-limits on SCD, Paleo diets allowed it if it was naturally sweetened and dairy-free.

The box listed sugar, marshmallows (sugar, corn syrup, modified cornstarch, gelatin, artificial flavor), corn syrup, modified whey, cocoa (processed with alkali), hydrogenated coconut oil, nonfat milk, calcium carbonate, less than 2 percent of salt, dipotassium phosphate, mono- and diglycerides, carrageenan, acesulfame.

I didn't even know how to pronounce some of those things, but I knew sugar, corn, and milk were out, so into the donate pile it went. I made a mental note to research some of the less familiar words later.

Surely the can of garden vegetable soup had to be healthy. I turned the can over and read "water, potatoes, carrots, tomato puree, tomatoes, corn, celery, kidney beans, green beans, modified food starch, salt, sugar, potassium chloride, corn protein (hydrolyzed), natural flavor, citric acid, calcium chloride, yeast extract."

Because of the potatoes, corn, and kidney beans, I couldn't keep this either. But why did they put modified anything into soup? And sugar? And what did *hydrolyzed* mean? I remembered reading that citric acid usually came from potatoes or corn. And yeast was on my food allergy list. I had to wait until my towheaded toddler finished building his skyscraper tower of cans before adding it to the giveaway pile.

Panko bread crumbs and regular Italian bread crumbs were next. *Wheat flour.* Nope. *Cane sugar.* Another no-no. *Yeast, salt.* No and yes. The only thing in the box I could eat was the salt.

Ryan's favorite brand of potato chips was next under the

microscope. Chips had to be benign, right? Or at least clean enough that we could keep them as a treat?

The ingredient list was a long one: "Dried potatoes, vegetable oil (corn, cottonseed, high oleic soybean, and/or sunflower oil), degerminated yellow corn flour, cornstarch, rice flour, maltodextrin, mono- and diglycerides. Contains 2% or less of salt, whey, sour cream (cream, nonfat milk, cultures), monosodium glutamate, onion powder, coconut oil, dextrose, sugar, natural flavors, nonfat milk, citric acid, sodium caseinate, lactic acid, yeast extract, disodium inosinate, disodium guanylate, buttermilk, malic acid, invert sugar, cultured nonfat milk, cream, wheat starch." Once again, I googled unfamiliar ingredients and realized several were inflammatory, were processed or made with chemicals, or had a high glycemic index.

With each chuck to the donate pile, I grew more and more frustrated at what seemed to be the sneakiness of the food industry. *Why put soy, corn, wheat, maltodextrin, MSG, and the sweetener dextrose in potato chips? Isn't the potato enough on its own?*

I consoled myself with the knowledge that a hundred dollars' worth of groceries was a drop in the bucket compared to the past four years' medical expenses. Even with insurance, some of the prescriptions alone dwarfed our weekly food allowance. And I reminded myself that I would *much* rather spend time in the kitchen cooking from scratch than in bed or at the hospital—*or in the bathroom.*

No, I reassured myself. *This is good. You're doing the right thing.* Then I got to the freezer. When I pulled out the half gallon of Thrifty Chocolate Malted Krunch ice cream and set it on the counter, I almost cried. It was my grandma Bonnie's special treat for us every time we would visit or spend the night at her house, and she had passed away right after Asher was born. But I knew my weaknesses. I also knew I was one of the best rationalizers on the planet. If it was in the house, not only would I eat it, I'd come up with a world-class excuse for why it was somehow okay. Well, not anymore. Any temptation—no matter how small or "innocent"—had to go. *That means you, sweet friend*, I said, placing a pint of mint chocolate chip ice cream on the counter next to the Chocolate Malted Krunch.

The only exception I allowed was if the box or something in the fridge or freezer was already opened. If it was perishable and couldn't be gifted to someone else (in fairness, I had stuck many spoons directly into those ice cream cartons for a quick bite), Ryan could finish it. Everything else was bagged and donated to neighbors, local food banks, or the people at Ryan's office.

Now that the kitchen was practically bare, it was time to restock. So I printed a list of foods I was allowed to have along with a few recipes I'd found online, bundled up Asher, and headed to the grocery store.

I spent most of my time shopping along the perimeter of the store—namely, in the produce and meat sections—as opposed to the aisles themselves, where all the canned, prepackaged, and heavily processed foods were located. I also diverted my attention from the endcaps, filled to the brim with the tempting and addicting foods I could no longer have.

I pushed my shopping cart into the produce area, where a rainbow of colorful fresh fruits and vegetables greeted me. But even there, I knew I needed to be discerning. I couldn't just grab a cucumber, bell pepper, pear, or bag of spinach because I knew that some of them could potentially have a film of insecticides, waxes, and other chemicals, none of which were good for the gut.

Instead, I walked straight to the smaller, pricier organic section and filled my cart with all the fruits and vegetables I loved—yellow bananas, tart apples, green leafy lettuces, fuzzy peaches, and green, globe-shaped artichokes with their prickly leaves—all of them herbicide-, pesticide-, and GMO-free. Asher loved strawberries and blueberries, so I threw in a few containers and moved on to the bulk nut section.

"See, Asher?" I said, handing him a beautiful, bright red bell pepper on the way. "No ingredient list. What you see is what you get. Just real food."

I bypassed the bakery, holding my breath so I wouldn't be tempted by the smell of all the yeasty baked goodness, and headed to the meat section, making sure to pick up only pasture-raised chicken, grass-fed and pasture-raised beef, and wild (not farm-raised) fish. I swallowed hard as I looked at the prices.

You would think that allowing the cows to roam freely and feed off the natural land would be cheaper and easier for the farmers, but I had learned that it actually takes a lot more work. For one thing, grass-fed farms have smaller herd sizes so the farmers can give the animals the attention they need. And in order for the herd to get the nutrients they need, the farmers have to move them to different pastures throughout the day, allowing the previously grazed pasture time to regrow. Also, the farmers have to select grasses that will nourish the cows best, so they are constantly planting new grass to supplement what naturally grows in the fields. This is referred to as managed grazing, and while it's definitely healthier for the cows— and for the people who eat their beef and drink their milk—it's also a lot more time-consuming and expensive for the farmers. Hence the higher price tag. I found out that the same basic rules apply to pasture-raised chicken and wild salmon, both of which require smaller groupings, more open space, and healthier diets in order to produce the healthiest stock.

"Happy, healthy chickens make happy, healthy people," I cooed to Asher as I placed a tray of plump pasture-raised, organic chicken breasts in the cart. *Why are they smaller than the regular ones I used to buy?* Then I realized . . . no steroids. I knew buying a whole chicken, bone in and skin on, would be more cost-efficient, but I just wasn't there

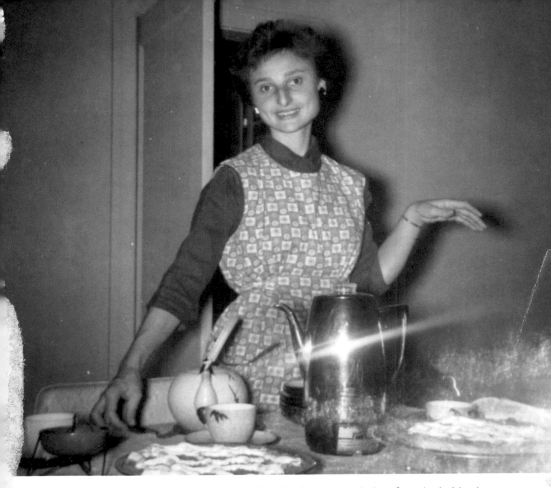

My grandma Marge in 1958, doing what she loves most in her favorite habitat!

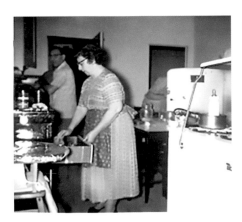

My dad's grandparents, Granny Sarella & Grandpa Michael, prep for a typical extended family Italian gathering in Oakland in 1956

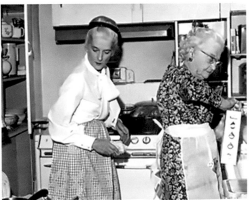

My great-grandma (on my dad's side), Ruby, and her mom, Ruby Darling, preparing the family's 1958 Thanksgiving dinner in Los Angeles

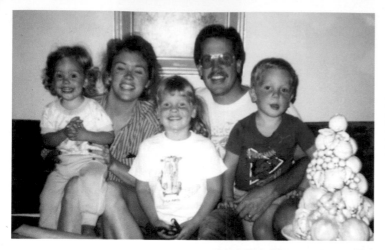

My parents, Cindi and Bob, in 1987 with us kids: me (on Mom's lap), Leisa, and Joel

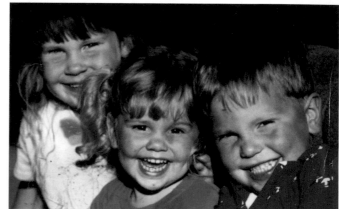

Me (center) & my siblings when I was about three in 1988

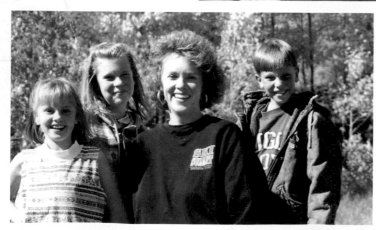

Me, Leisa, Mom & Joel in Aspen

My family traveling through Europe in 1999 to celebrate my sister's high school graduation

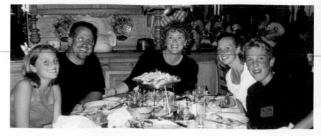

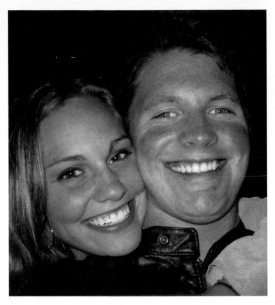

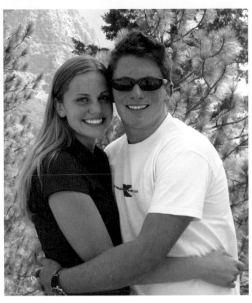

Date night with Ryan at a steak house

Our trip to Yosemite to camp with friends in celebration of Ryan's 2002 high school graduation

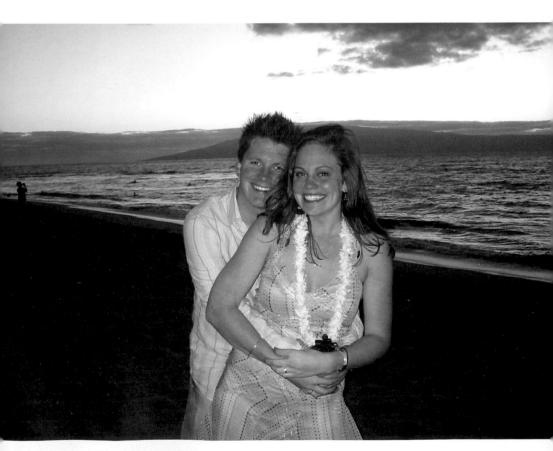

Our engagement in Maui, Hawaii, in 2005

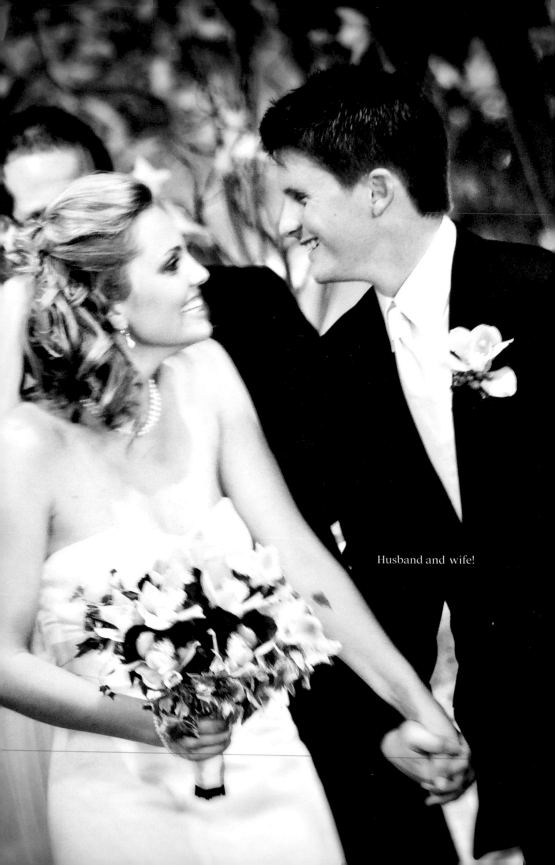

Husband and wife!

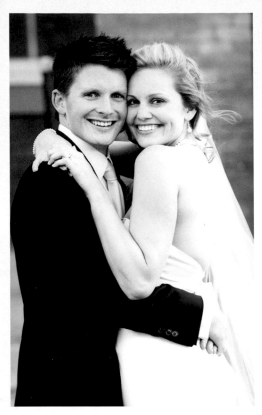

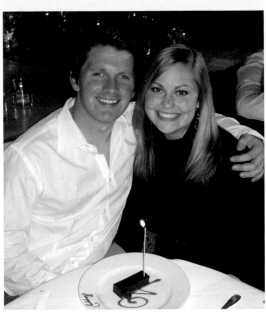

Celebrating our first anniversary
in San Francisco

Our wedding day in 2007 at the Presidio,
a former military base in San Francisco

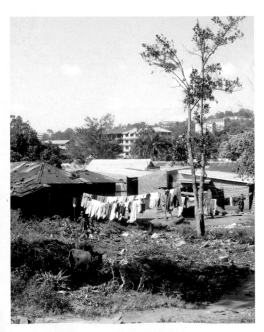

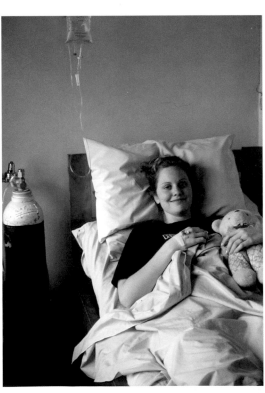

The drive through Kampala
to the hospital

My hospital room in Kampala, Uganda, in 2008.
One of the little girls on our team, Annie,
sent her teddy bear to comfort me.
She never went anywhere without that bear.

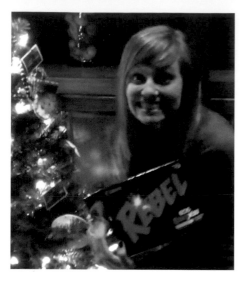

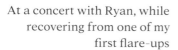

Ryan surprised me in 2009 with my first camera—the Canon Rebel—that I used to take photos for my first cookbooks.

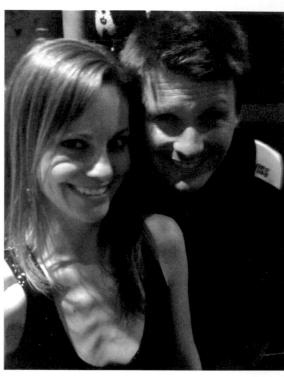

At a concert with Ryan, while recovering from one of my first flare-ups

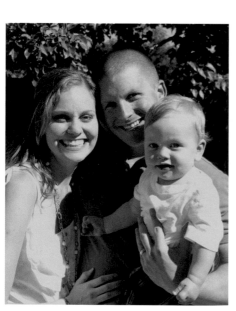

Back home with Ryan & Asher for Father's Day 2011 after my flare-up and long hospitalization

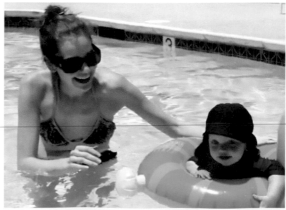

Swimming at our community pool with Asher after my hospitalization in 2011. I had lost thirty pounds in the previous two weeks.

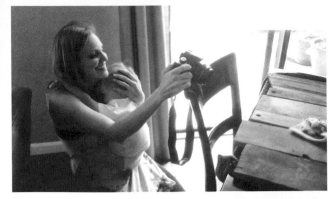

Photographing my Real-Deal Chocolate-Chip Cookies for the first time. I tried to take photos during Asher's naps, but on this day he had other plans.

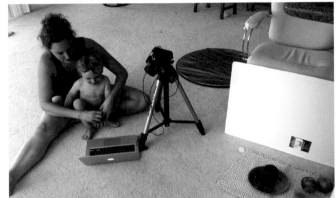

Photographing recipes in Kona, Hawaii, for my first cookbook, *Against All Grain*

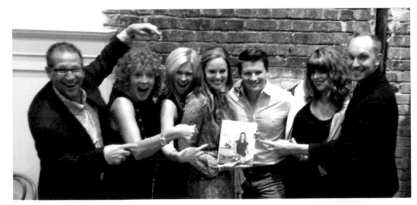

My family celebrating the release of *Against All Grain* in 2013

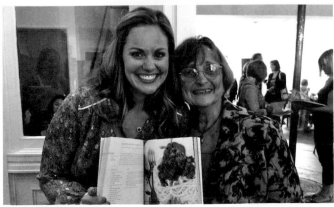

Showing off Granny Sarella's spaghetti sauce recipe in *Against All Grain* with her daughter, Grandma Marge

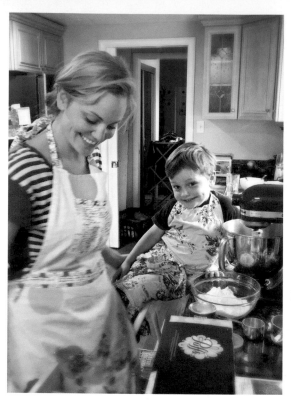

Baking with three-year-old Asher

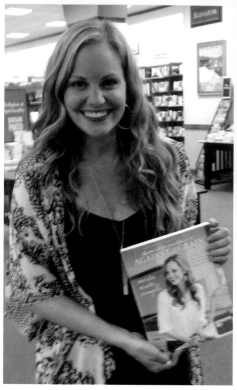

Capping off a date night with Ryan
by stopping at Barnes & Noble
to find a copy of the just-released
Meals Made Simple

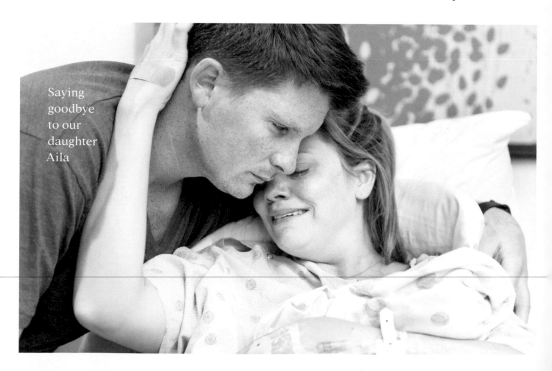

Saying
goodbye
to our
daughter
Aila

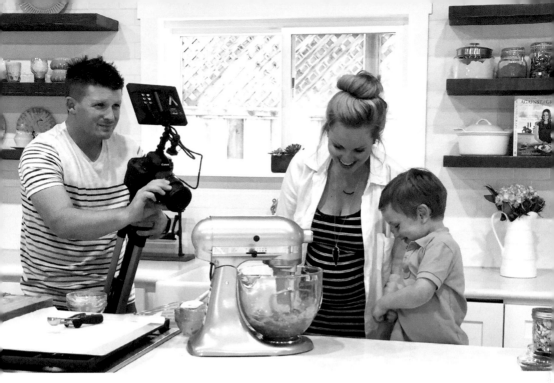

Ryan films a YouTube episode of Asher making cookies
with me while I was pregnant with Easton.

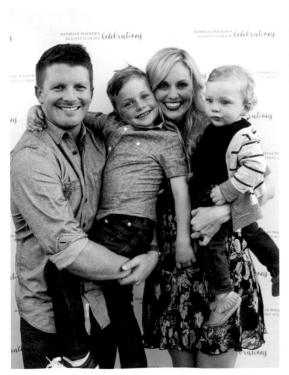

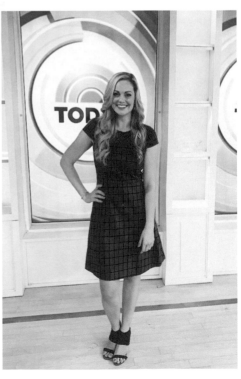

Marking the release of *Celebrations* at
the Sideboard café in Lafayette, CA

My first *Today* show appearance to
celebrate the 2016 release of *Celebrations*

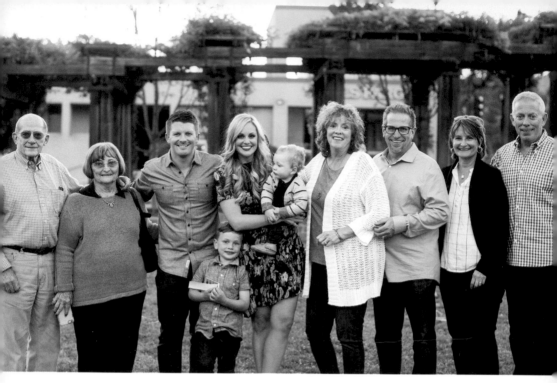

Commemorating the release of *Celebrations* in 2016 with (from left)
Grandpa Wynn and Grandma Marge; Ryan, Asher, and me holding Easton;
my parents, Cindi and Bob; and Ryan's parents, Barb and Dwight

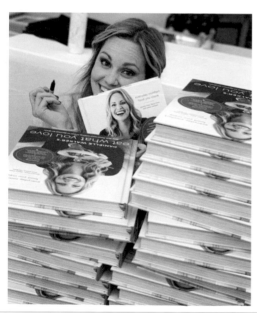

I signed 400 copies of *Eat What You Love*
each night during my 2018 book tour!

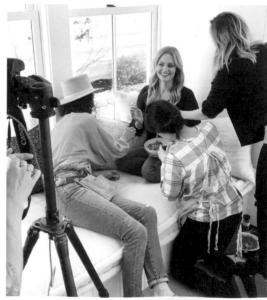

Behind the scenes of the cover
shoot for *Eat What You Love*

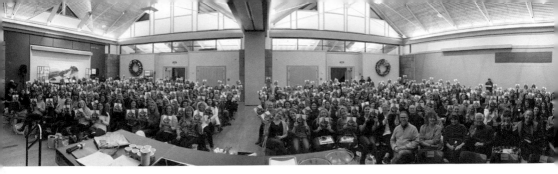

The wonderful crowd waiting for my appearance at an *Eat What You Love* release event

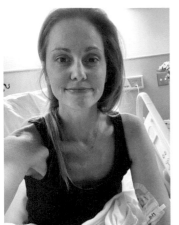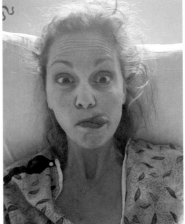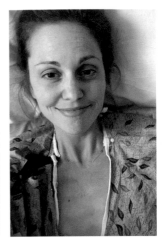

In 2019, I was rushed to the hospital after an extreme flare-up.
I took selfies for Ryan and the kids to let them know I was going to be okay.

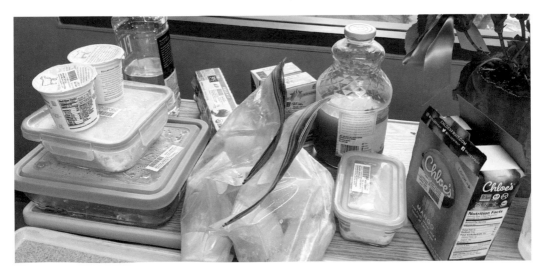

My hospital food! A kind nurse kept it in the fridge for me so I had an alternative
to the hospital food, which could have made my flare-up even worse.

FaceTiming with Kezia
from my hospital bed
while she downed
Chipotle guacamole

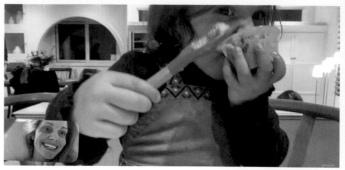

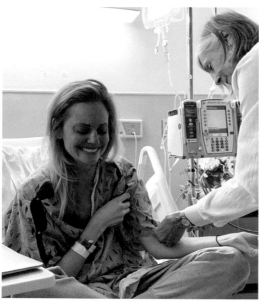

Removing my PICC line
so I could go to the courtyard

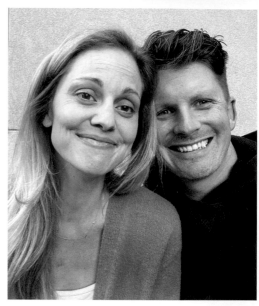

Breaking free from my hospital room
and waiting to see my babies

A precious
visit with my
kids for the
first time
in 12 days

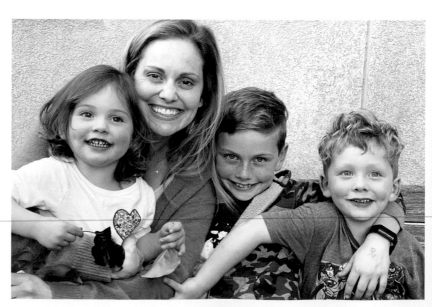

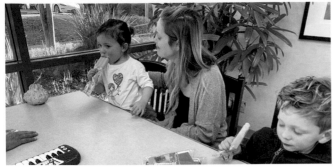

My second time visiting with the kids during my three-week hospital stay. We made crafts and had popsicles in the cafeteria to have some normalcy. I was exhausted after twenty minutes.

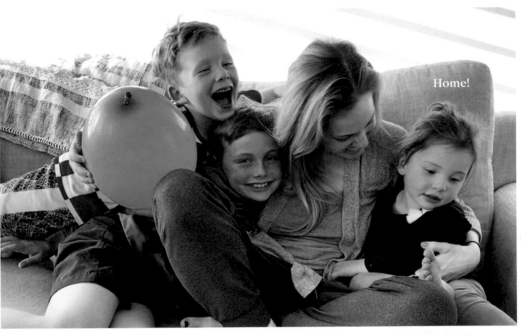

Home!

Thanksgiving 2019, just a few days after returning home. My only job was to cut up the Nut-Free Lunch-Box Bread from *Eat What You Love* for the stuffing—and boss my mom and mother-in-law around the kitchen from my stool.

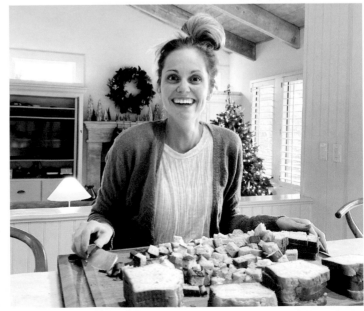

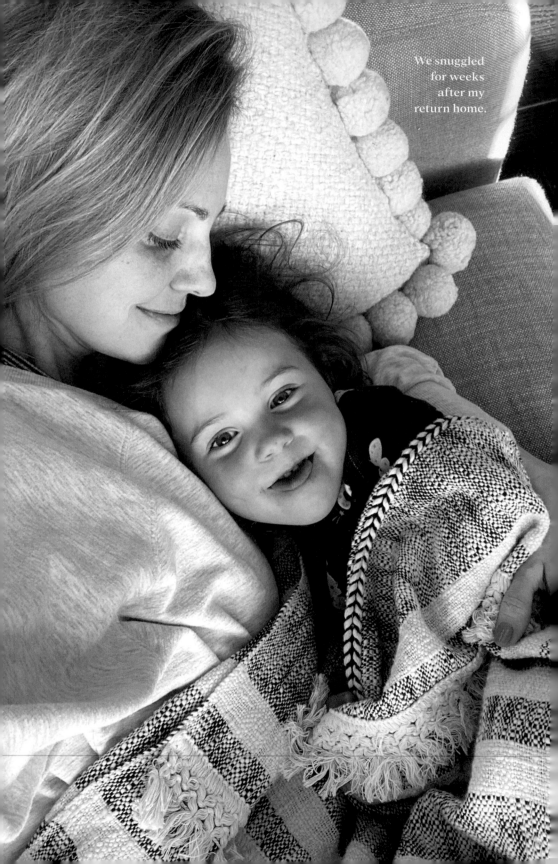

We snuggled
for weeks
after my
return home.

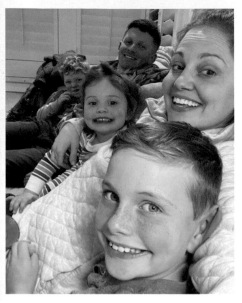

A quiet 2019 New Year's Eve
on the couch with my family

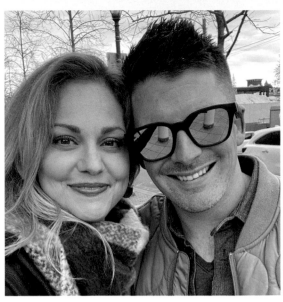

First date night out after my hospitalization.
My cheeks were just starting to puff up
from the prednisone.

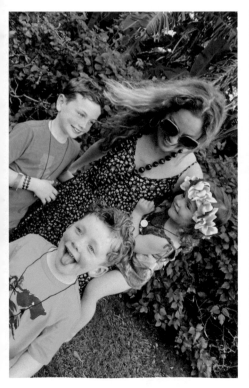

Enjoying a luau—and pretending
we are Disney's Moana all night

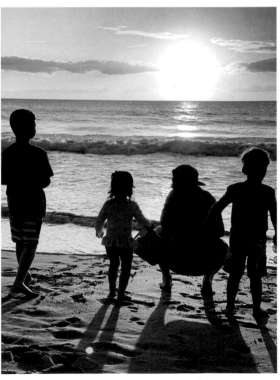

The sunset in Maui in early 2020

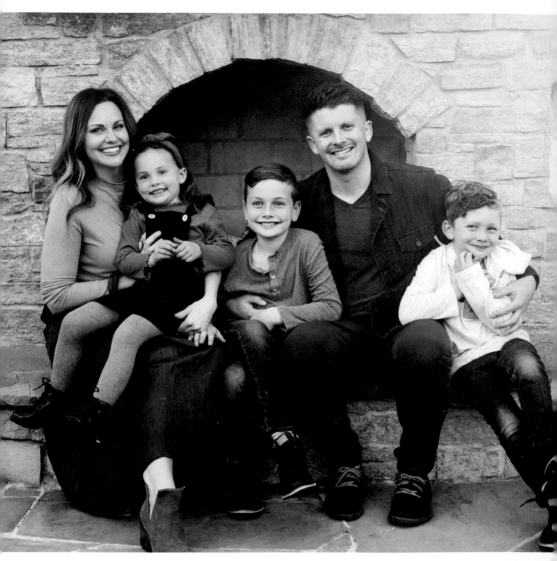

Our family, March 2021. Kezia (3), Asher (10), Easton (5).

yet. In my past life I had used frozen chicken so I wouldn't have to handle the slimy raw meat.

I moved on to the eggs and found a carton labeled pasture-raised, organic, and soy-free. They were twice the price of the brand I normally bought, but I chanted in my head over and over that this was going to save us money in the end.

Once I'd stocked up on beef, chicken, and salmon, I cautiously made my way into the aisles. I started at the baby snacks aisle because Asher was getting restless and had lost interest in that red bell pepper. Instead of my usuals, I grabbed a few packages of the better-for-you alternatives that said *organic* and *nothing artificial* and threw them into my cart. I snatched one and quickly gave it to Asher in hopes of holding his attention while I finished flipping and dissecting packages.

I picked up a jar of "natural" almond butter, which I was now allowed to eat again, and turned the jar around so I could read the ingredient list. *Almonds, canola oil, cane sugar . . . Why do they need to add cane sugar and canola oil to something "natural"?* I sighed and put the jar back on the shelf. Once I found a jar containing almonds and salt only, I added it to the heap.

With each item, I had the same routine: pick it up, turn it over, read the ingredient list to determine if it contained anything that wasn't good for my body, then either return it to the shelf or place it in my cart. And it wasn't easy. It turns out that gluten wasn't the only thing that could hide out under another name. Maltodextrin, for example, which shows up in everything from soup mixes and salad dressings to those "potato" chips I had at home, is made from corn, potatoes, rice, or even sometimes wheat. Likewise, dextrose is another name for sugar. Monosodium glutamate is MSG. Xanthan gum can be cross-contaminated with wheat and is hard to digest; rapeseed oil is actually canola oil, neither of which I could have because they were highly processed and high in omega-6 fatty acids, which could increase inflammation.

Even the things touted as healthy alternatives were problematic. Agave nectar, for instance, was heavily processed and had an even higher fructose content than table sugar. And carrageenan, a "natural" thickener used in almond and coconut milk, is made from seaweed but is also a known gut irritant.

I laughed when I saw *Gluten-free!* marketed on a bag of potato chips. I know I was still learning the ins and outs of gluten myself, but it was such a buzzword that the term was even put on bottled water to get people's attention. Clearly gluten shouldn't be in potato chips or bottled water. I started to be thankful for marketing words that prompted me to check the ingredients.

I grabbed a few cans of full-fat, 100 percent coconut milk (not the cartons because they had binders and stabilizers) and a few jarred tomato sauces that were free of citric acid, soybean oil, and sugar. A big bottle of extra-virgin olive oil and a jar of unrefined snow-white coconut oil would replace the sticky yellow plastic bottle of oil I had tossed out. I also selected a jar of raw, creamy honey from the shelf next to the almond butter. I was hoping to find bags of almond flour in the baking section, but they only had all-purpose, gluten-free blends, and whole-wheat flour. I guessed I would have to visit a health-food store for that, or maybe order it online.

By the time my cart was full, Asher was getting cranky and fidgety and had devoured his rice teething stick. "Oh my gosh," I said checking my watch. "We've been here for almost two hours and it's well past your nap time!"

I quickly pushed my overflowing cart to the checkout lane and braced myself for the sticker shock. *Okay,* I reminded myself as the cashier swiped one item after another across the belt, *restocking an entire pantry is going to be expensive—the first time. But I won't have to keep buying all this stuff every time I come to the store. A lot of these things will last for a long time.* When the final total flashed across the screen I almost blacked out. *What is Ryan going to say?* Then I looked down at Asher and smiled. I knew he would tell me, "You can't put a price tag on your health, Danielle. And it's a lot cheaper than spending a week in the hospital or paying eight hundred dollars a month for medications."

Fortunately, Asher had already started to doze off in his car seat on the way home, because I had *a ton* of groceries to unload, and the thought of trying to do it while wearing a baby sling was not appealing. After I got Asher unbuckled and settled into his crib for a nap, I started to unpack the car. Within no time, the countertops were covered with grain-free, gluten-free, dairy-free, sugar-free, fresh, organic, grass-fed goodness. *Okay*, I thought, surveying the scene. *Now that I have all this stuff, what do I do with it?* Candidly, it was a little overwhelming. A lot overwhelming.

———————

The lists told me what to buy and why. What they didn't tell me, however, was how to take that chicken breast, bell pepper, coconut oil, organic honey, apple cider vinegar, and ghee (clarified butter), and turn it all into an edible dinner for two. I glanced at my watch—*in under an hour!*

I suddenly felt exhausted. *Maybe I should just order takeout.*

No. You can do this. Just start simple, I told myself, reaching for the chicken breasts. My mom frequently made stir-fry with whatever we had left in the fridge at the end of the week, so I started there. Although without soy sauce and cornstarch, I wasn't exactly sure how to do that. *You can figure out the actual recipes later.* That night, Ryan and I had a simple, inflammation-friendly stir-fry of chicken rubbed in curry powder, ginger, and cumin, to which I added a little coconut milk to make a curry sauce of sorts. I sautéed a side of mixed veggies in coconut oil and seasoned them with sea salt.

God bless Ryan. He ate every last bite and didn't even flinch when he noticed that his beloved white rice was missing from the plate. Or when he glanced at the ridiculously high grocery receipt I'd left out on the counter. While I appreciated his patience, given what I had just spent, I had no intention of serving that poor man only chicken and veggies for the rest of his life. *At least he'll be able to finish off what's left of the ice cream for dessert*, I thought.

I knew I could pull together some simple steak and fish dishes to get me through the first week or so while I looked for more recipes and figured out how to use all this stuff. I thought it would be nice to have some kind of homemade dessert—especially now that the ice cream was gone. I wanted something to give Ryan—and myself—hope that better meals were on the horizon.

I pulled out my bridal shower index cards again. *Hmm . . . it's getting close to the holidays*, I thought, flipping through the stack. *Pumpkin pie! Perfect.* I looked over the ingredients. The pumpkin filling part was easy—the pumpkin and the spices could remain the same. I just couldn't use the can of Libby's Easy Pumpkin Pie Mix my mom used, which included the pumpkin, sugar, milk, and spices all in one. *I need just plain and simple pumpkin puree. And I'll switch out the sugar for maple syrup and use almond milk instead of regular.*

The crust was a little trickier. I didn't want a bland crust. This was a traditional holiday pie—all of it had to taste perfect! My mom always bought premade crusts or pie dough, so I did a quick search online for the highest-rated pie dough. All-purpose flour, salt, shortening or butter, and ice water. *What if I just use almond flour instead of regular?*

I knew from the banana muffin recipe that it wasn't going to be a one-to-one ratio, so I guesstimated, playing with the flour and oil combination, tweaking it a little bit at a time until I finally landed on substituting one and three-quarters cups of almond flour and one-third cup of coconut oil instead of the cubes of butter my grandmother used to cut in. For my sugar substitute, I tried honey. *There, that oughta do it*, I thought, reviewing the original recipe. *No sugar. No wheat flour. No vegetable oil or butter.* Then I added the usual vanilla, salt, baking soda, and a bit of ground cinnamon and ginger, mixed all the ingredients together until they were just combined, and then pressed the dough into a pie plate.

It didn't look exactly like pie dough; it was a little oilier and crumblier. But it was close. I prebaked the crust as usual. Despite its original non-doughy consistency, it held together nicely and actually looked like it was supposed to. The question was, would it *taste* like it was supposed to? And would it cut into clean slices once the filling was baked in it? I pinched a bit off the edge, popped it into my mouth, and held my breath. *Not bad! Not bad at all, in fact.*

While the crust cooled on the counter, I turned my attention to the filling. I whisked all the ingredients together in a bowl, smiling as I watched the rich pumpkin turn the entire filling a deep autumn orange. As I poured it over the piecrust, I found myself licking my lips in anticipation. I couldn't wait to try it. After about thirty minutes, I inserted a toothpick into the center, and it came out with just a tiny bit of the filling clinging to it. I pushed it back into the oven and closed the door, counting the minutes until I could pull it out. When I checked again, the center was set and slightly jiggly, so I removed it from the oven, placed it on the counter, and stood back to evaluate it. It looked the same as regular pumpkin pie. But how would it taste? I dropped my fork into it and took a bite. *Oh, wow.* I took another bite. *All this needs is some whipped cream and it will be perfect!*

Whipped cream . . . hmm. I can't have real dairy cream anymore. And I'm guessing those cans of aerosol whipped cream we used to squirt straight into our mouths as kids weren't solely cream anyway.

I did a quick search on dairy-free whipped cream and saw a few blogs that sang the praises of coconut milk whipped cream. I had noticed the thick cream on the tops of the cans I had opened to make curry or to use in some of my baking experiments, but I'd never thought to whip it up!

There was only one problem: All the blogs said you had to refrigerate the can for at least twenty-four hours. All of mine were in the pantry. And in the California heat, they were nowhere near cold.

Next time, I resolved. *It's pretty good on its own.* What I would have given, though, to grab some cold vanilla ice cream out of the freezer and make it à la mode.

The pumpkin pie a resounding success, I turned my attention to soups and sides. Because each recipe I tried required so many tweaks to get the taste and consistency just right, I started keeping my own recipe journal. I recorded all the ingredients I used, how I tweaked each version, and the results I got from each attempt (good and bad).

Whenever Asher napped, I went online and researched the science behind cooking and baking. I loved *Cook's Illustrated* and *America's Test Kitchen* because they broke down why certain things worked and others didn't. And I especially loved reading Alton Brown's recipes because he often went into the science behind the ingredients and the methods he used to explain why a soufflé would rise, what made a cookie crispy, or what putting a bowl of water in the oven could do for a loaf of bread (spoiler alert—the steam helps the crust crisp up and the center rise).

Even when I couldn't use the recipes, which was 95 percent of the time, I still read for the knowledge to help me find substitutes. For example, I wanted to understand why some recipes used white sugar while others called for brown sugar or molasses. What I learned was that when melted, granulated sugar reacts much differently than honey or maple syrup, which are already liquids. So if I wanted to add a little bit of crunch to a recipe, granulated sugar—or, in my case, a healthier sub of coconut sugar—would be helpful.

Some recipes were easy to convert, like Granny Sarella's spaghetti sauce. All I really had to do was switch to grass-fed beef and swap out the sugar for honey. I served it over shredded spaghetti squash or zucchini pulled through a julienne slicer to make long noodles.

Other dishes took a little more time and experimentation to get "just right," like Grandma Bonnie's sour meatballs. I could swap in some almond flour for the crackers, but the texture was quite different and it didn't make the meatballs as soft and tender. And I still wasn't sure how to thicken a gravy without the use of a flour and butter roux or a cornstarch slurry, which was my dad's tactic at Thanksgiving.

Unfortunately, Mom's shepherd's pie proved impossible to recreate without all the canned creamy soups and dairy products. And it just wasn't the same without those crunchy fried onions on top.

Without question, however, the biggest disaster was the macaroni and cheese I tried to make for Asher. I started by soaking raw cashews in water to soften them and then blending them into a creamy sauce. Then I took some nutritional yeast, which the internet claimed tasted like cheese, and combined it with the cashews. The sauce finished, I turned my attention to the pasta. I often ran vegetables like zucchini or butternut squash through a spiralizer machine to make noodles, but neither the shape nor the texture were quite right for mac and cheese. *What about cauliflower?* As I grabbed a head of cauliflower from the crisper, I flashed back to the disastrous runny mashed-potato substitute I'd made for Thanksgiving. It was bad enough I'd had to eat that sloppy mess. There was no way I was going to subject poor Asher to it.

I looked at the simple white florets all bunched together like a cloud. *The stalks are kind of chewy,* I reasoned. *Maybe if I just used those and didn't cook them all the way . . . that should give me a chewy-like pasta.* It sounded good in my head, so I cut the stalks up into little macaroni-like pieces, blanched them in hot water, folded them into the sauce, and then helped myself to a steaming forkful. It tasted—in a word—awful.

Maybe if I add a little salt, I thought optimistically. I tried it again and almost gagged. *Don't panic*, I thought, frantically scouring the fridge for a solution. *Maybe a little lemon juice or apple cider vinegar to add a bit of a cheesy zing?* I tried both. If anything, that made it even more inedible. In fact, it was hard to tell which was worse, the cauliflower "noodles" that tasted nothing like pasta or the sauce that, if I'm being honest, both smelled and *tasted*—I expect—like stinky feet.

Because eating healthy was so expensive, normally we ate everything I made, even the failures. But this stuff . . . *I can't put them through this.* And with that, I dumped the entire bowl into the trash.

Fortunately, that was my worst experiment. For the most part, the more I learned about the science of food and what flavors work well together, the fewer test versions it took before my creations came out tasting the way I'd hoped. The macaroni and cheese disaster aside, a little extra seasoning or splash of citrus usually did the trick.

But it wasn't enough for *me* to like it. Any time I tried a new recipe, I tested it on Ryan, my grandma, my neighbors, or my parents. And I didn't give them any disclaimers first, like "This is grain-free" or "This is dairy-free." I simply said, "Hey, I made cashew chicken for dinner" or "I think you'll love this chocolate mousse." Then I'd wait to hear their reactions before telling them what was missing—or, in some cases, what I'd put in it (like the avocados I used in my chocolate mousse). I wanted their honest feedback, so after every meal, I would ask them a series of questions to gauge if a recipe was worthy of being published on my blog:

Did you notice that there were no grains or dairy?
Was the texture okay?
Do you think it needs more spices? More salt?
Should it have been cooked longer?
Is it sweet enough?
Is the crumb of the muffin similar enough to a regular gluten-
    filled muffin?

My dad hates avocados and devoured the mousse without so much as a cringe, so I knew that one was a winner.

The one thing I couldn't seem to master was pasta, which drove me crazy. I had always loved lasagna, and I was determined to come up with something that tasted as good as Grandma Marge's.

I tried slicing zucchini into long, flat sheets, but they sweat so much during the cooking process that the bottom of the casserole dish was literally pooling with water. I started salting the zucchini and letting it sweat on paper towels, which helped a lot with the moisture, and then I began breading it in an egg wash and almond flour with seasonings. That made the texture more similar to noodles. But it still tasted like a vegetable, and it was a long, tedious process to add to the already tedious lasagna-making process.

Maybe vegetables aren't the way to go. I flipped through my recipe journal, stopping on a coconut-flour crepe I'd been working on for sandwich wraps and to wrap around almond butter and bananas in the mornings. *Maybe that could work for the pasta layers.* I had used them for enchiladas and they held up to the sauce and fillings. It was worth a shot.

I made a dozen thin crepes using the egg, almond milk, coconut flour, and coconut oil mixture I'd perfected. I then set them aside to concentrate on the cheese. There was no way I was going anywhere near nutritional yeast for the foreseeable future. In addition to tasting terrible, the texture was totally wrong. I opened the refrigerator to see what I had available. *There has to be something dairy-free that mimics ricotta cheese.* My eyes settled on the large container of almond milk on the middle shelf. I had been making my own almond milk for months now and had been trying to think of some way to reuse the leftover pulp after I strained out the liquid. Now that I was thinking about it, the texture kind of reminded me of a dry ricotta. It didn't taste anything like cheese, but maybe I could add something to it to give it that zesty flavor that cheese has. It made sense. Cheese was made from milk. Almond milk tasted somewhat like milk. Wouldn't it stand to reason that you could get a cheese-like flavor from the same stuff you get almond milk from?

I grabbed a bag of almonds from the pantry and soaked them overnight the way I would to make milk. The next day instead of adding cups of water to thin it out in the blender, I added salt, a bit of water, extra-virgin olive oil, and lemon juice to create the home-made, slightly sour, cultured flavor of cheese. I had seen recipes in my old cookbooks calling for buttermilk and noting that adding lemon juice to milk could be substituted. Maybe my tweaks would have a similar effect? I reached my spoon into the food processor and tried a bit off the edge.

It wasn't bad. I added a little more salt and an extra splash of lemon juice, and *bingo*! If I just added a little tomato sauce and Italian seasoning, it would taste just like the real thing in my lasagna.

I pulled out a casserole dish and started building layers of crepes, cut into lasagna-sized strips, topped with crumbled Italian sausage, homemade marinara sauce, the almond ricotta, and fresh spinach. I then sprinkled the top with parsley, basil, salt, and pepper. It was even more labor-intensive than regular lasagna, but if it tasted similar, it would be worth every minute. Besides, if it worked, I could make two and keep one in the freezer to have on hand when I didn't have time to make something or friends came over unexpectedly. Same amount of dishes, half the work.

When the lasagna finally came out of the oven, the smell was amazing—pure Italian. And the way the sauce bubbled up around the edges of the crepes, smothering the still-sizzling sausage, lightly wilted spinach leaves, and crumbly white almond ricotta made it look exactly like the lasagna Grandma Marge made. It even resembled the Stouffer's one my mom always kept in our freezer.

The aroma was so delicious that it drew Ryan right out of the living room where he was playing with Ash and into the kitchen. "What smells so good in here?"

"I made lasagna," I said, a slight hint of pride in my voice.

Ryan glanced over my shoulder at the beautifully bubbling dish, his eyebrows raised in surprise. "Wow. That looks fantastic."

There's only one way to find out, I thought, grabbing a spatula. There weren't any stretchy strings of cheese lifting up from the pan when I pulled out a slice, but otherwise it perfectly mimicked the flavors and textures of the classic Italian dish I had always loved. Ryan even had a second helping.

Yes! Not only were we eating healthy, we were enjoying it!

10

"You're putting all these recipes on your blog, right?" Ryan asked, taking a bite of my Italian baked eggs.

"Oh my gosh! My blog!" I had completely forgotten about it. Back when I started it, right before Asher was born, I had only two or three recipes (and pretty basic ones at that), but now . . .

That week, I remade all my favorite recipes—the honey biscuits that reminded me of corn bread, cashew chicken, chicken Parmesan with spaghetti squash (it was cooked through this time!), SCD cupcakes with frosting, double-chocolate ice cream with almond butter swirl, apple spice coffee cake, and coconut-crusted chicken strips with honey mustard that I kept in my freezer to make easy lunches for Asher. I even made another lasagna (much to Ryan's delight). As soon as each dish came out of the oven, I plated up a piece and snapped pictures with my camera, choosing one or two to post alongside the recipe.

Most of the comments I received on the blog came courtesy of my mom, my sister, and my grandmother—all raves, of course. There was also one anonymous comment that I'm fairly certain came from Ryan to bolster my confidence. It sounded an awful lot like the sticky love notes he left on my bathroom mirror most mornings before he left for work. Other than that, nobody else seemed to know my blog existed. I just figured I'd keep posting recipes and maybe some-day someone with my condition might stumble across it and find it helpful. Until then, if nothing else, it inspired me to keep trying new recipes.

"So," Ryan asked one morning as I was uploading my latest recipe, "what's next?"

"Actually, I was thinking about trying a few more baked goods. Like those old banana muffins we used to eat a lot." I missed baked goods. Every time I went to the grocery store, I practically had to hold my breath walking past the bakery section to keep temp-tation at bay. The problem was, cooking was one thing; baking, which is all about using very specific amounts of specific ingredi-ents to create even more specific chemical reactions, was another. Except for my brief foray into banana muffins and peanut butter cookies, everything else I tried had literally fallen flat. Every grain-free cake and muffin recipe I found online always came out soggy and greasy. And for some reason, without fail, they all sank in the middle.

"Well, the timing couldn't be more perfect," he said, pulling Asher out of his high chair and into a big hug.

He was right about that. Fall was approaching, and my hereditary love of the holidays had me craving pumpkin bread like crazy. *I know I can eat pumpkin*, I thought, *and the pie went well. How much harder can a simple loaf be?* I took my recipe binder off the kitchen shelf and pulled out my mom's old go-to pumpkin bread recipe.

White sugar
Brown sugar
All-purpose flour
Baking powder

I laughed to myself. *Four for four. Okay, looks like we're starting from scratch.* I knew a one-to-one ratio with the flour ingredients wouldn't work, but I wasn't sure what the correct ratio should be, and with baking, there was no room for error. I'd already tried almond flour, and it was okay, but it had a greasy and gritty texture. Maybe that's why everything seemed to sink in the middle whenever I used it as the only flour. I started poking around in my pantry. *What about coconut flour?* I wondered, pulling out a bag. I had just recently started seeing it at the store, and I threw it into my cart during my last shopping trip because I knew I could eat coconut and the word *flour* intrigued me. But I'd never seen anyone bake with it online or explain how it should be used.

Because the coconut flour had the powdery consistency of all-purpose flour, I decided to start with a one-to-one substitution to see what happened. The recipe called for two cups of all-purpose flour, so I put two cups of coconut flour in. As soon as I added the wet ingredients, however, the flour sucked them up like a sponge. I decided to power through and see if it would magically change once it baked. The loaf came out of the oven like a brick—dense and disgusting.

My rule was to never throw things away, but this was inedible. After dropping it into the trash, I did a little digging online to find out what went wrong. I discovered that coconut flour is basically coconut that's been dehydrated and then ground into a fine powder. I had given Asher dehydrated apples before and watched as they seemed to come back to life when he decided to let them go swimming in his water cup. So I reasoned that I probably needed to use less coconut flour than the recipe called for to allow for rehydration. Half the flour? That didn't seem right, especially given how dense the coconut flour became. I thought for a minute. *If almond flour is too oily when it bakes and coconut flour is superabsorbent, what if I combine them?*

I'd read enough labels on store-bought gluten-free foods to see that they used a lot of flour blends—sometimes as many as three to six different flours and starches (rice, potato, corn, xanthan gum) to make up for the loss of gluten. Clearly, different gluten-free flours and starches reacted in different ways and worked together harmoniously to create that all-purpose wheat flour texture. I just needed to figure out which ones played well together.

Before digging back into my expensive cache of ingredients, I decided to go online to see if anybody else was trying different flour combinations. If so, I might save myself a little time and money. Surprisingly, I couldn't find anyone who was. *Am I the only one trying this?* A few more clicks of the mouse convinced me I was. I found recipes for muffins made solely with almond flour or ground pecans or walnuts. I saw others made solely with coconut flour. But I found none that used multiple flour substitutes. That was all the motivation I needed.

I spent the rest of the afternoon slowly adding coconut flour, one teaspoon at a time, to a base of almond flour, and stirring that into a mixture of fresh pumpkin puree, honey, coconut oil, eggs, and a blend of autumnal spices. The first loaf was still too oily. The second loaf was better, but still sank a bit in the middle. But the third loaf . . .

"Ryan!" I called out in excitement. "Come taste this!"

As soon as he popped a piece of the bread infused with cardamom, cinnamon, ginger, and nutmeg into his mouth, I knew.

Nailed it!

"Dan, this is awesome!" Ryan exclaimed, breaking off another piece. "How'd you do it?"

"It was the coconut flour," I said. "Up until now, I'd just been using almond flour, and that's why everything kept coming out so greasy and sunken down in the center. I realized the reason when I roasted almonds for our salad the other night. They release oil when heated. That's why everything I've baked has been greasy. But coconut flour absorbs the wet ingredients better and—" I stopped and stared at Ryan.

"What?" he mumbled, his mouth still full.

"Helps it hold its shape!" *That's it!* I reached up, grabbed Ryan's cheeks, and pulled him in for an enthusiastic kiss. "Can you keep an eye on Asher for a little while?"

"Sure," he said, a quizzical look on his face. "Why? What are you going to do?"

I reached into the pantry, pulled out what was left of my coconut flour, and then turned and smiled confidently at Ryan. "Make real bread."

I missed bread. Oh, how I missed bread. I missed grilled panini-style sandwiches; hot, buttered rolls; chewy pizza dough; and thick, egg-battered French toast covered in fresh, ripe berries. The problem was, no matter how hard I tried, I simply could not get grain-free, gluten-free bread to taste—or more importantly, feel—like bread.

"Again?" he asked, as I continued pulling ingredients out of the pantry. "I thought you said it didn't work." He was right. I'd tried multiple recipes, but without gluten, every loaf I made was either too crumbly, falling apart as soon as I took it out of the pan, or too dense, sinking in the middle. And those were their good points. In fact, we had a freezer full of inedible bread loaves. The ingredients were just so expensive I couldn't bring myself to throw them away. I figured I could crumble them into a casserole or make bread pudding at some point.

"It didn't," I said, taking some eggs out of the fridge. "But that was before I figured out how coconut flour works."

Ryan smiled and shook his head. By now he was used to me tearing the kitchen apart in a frenzy of baking madness. "Okay if I take the rest of this with me?" he asked, holding up the remainder of the pumpkin loaf and walking back toward Asher in the living room.

"It's all yours," I replied with a smile.

All right, I thought, *let's do this*. I picked up my recipe journal and flipped over to the section that documented my forays into bread making. Four full pages of failures. *I bet anything it's the flour.*

Convinced my wet ingredients weren't the culprit, I took four large eggs, separated the yolks and the whites, and beat the egg whites in my stand mixer until they formed soft peaks.

I had seen a few cake recipes online that claimed folding the whites in separately helped keep the mixture light and airy, which made perfect sense to me. I had made meringue cookies before, and those billowy pillows of sweetness were definitely airy. I think the almond flour was just too dense for the egg whites to overcome. And in order for me to get the texture of the almond flour smooth enough to mimic bread, I had been pureeing it in the food processor. That process probably deflated the whites every time.

In the pantry I found some cashew butter that I had used in choc-olate truffles and thought it might work in place of the almond flour. Cashews were a little more neutral in their taste. Also, this butter was already smooth, so it required no processing, and I knew from roasting nuts that cashews seemed to be less oily than almonds.

In a separate bowl, I beat the egg yolks together with some raw, unsweetened cashew butter. Then I added in some honey and a tiny splash of apple cider vinegar (to react with the baking soda and help it rise even more—like the volcano science experiments of my elemen-tary days). Finally, I added some almond milk and mixed it all together.

Then I turned my attention to the dry ingredients. "Here we go," I said, sifting the coconut flour together with a teaspoon of baking soda and a pinch of sea salt. *A quarter of a cup ought to do it*, I thought, remembering how quickly the coconut rehydrated during the baking process. Then I poured in the wet mixture and carefully folded in the beaten egg whites. *The amount looks about right*, I thought, eyeing the bowl. It looked more like a thick cake batter than a dough, but grain-free baking seemed to be that way, especially with coconut flour before it started its absorption process. Then I poured the batter into a loaf pan greased with coconut oil, said a quick prayer, and slid it into the oven.

For the next forty-five minutes, I was about as impatient as I've ever been in my life. Fortunately, between the pumpkin loaf and the great white bread experiment, I had made quite a mess in the kitchen, so at least I had the cleanup to distract me. When the oven timer finally went off, I opened the door and was immediately met with the unmistakable scent of . . . wait for it . . . freshly baked bread! It had even risen above the edges of the loaf pan. *That smells amazing*, I thought, sticking a toothpick in the center to see if it was done. *Yep—clean!* I pulled the glass pan out of the oven and slid a knife gently around the sides of the loaf to free it. Then I flipped the pan upside down and released the loaf onto a cooling rack.

It looked good. The crust was golden brown, and it was a lot taller than all my failed loaves. Most importantly, it was holding its shape. *I think it worked!* I was as giddy as a kid on Christmas morning, and it was all I could do to keep from slicing right into it. I had learned from the pumpkin loaf, however, that coconut flour needed to cool completely before I sliced it so the moisture could redistribute itself evenly throughout the loaf. If I cut into it too soon, it would be soggy and spongy.

Finally, after an hour-long wait that felt like a year, I grabbed a bread knife and slowly began to slice into it. The outside was slightly crusty, and the inside didn't disintegrate into a crumbly mess! My heart was beating at the rate of a hummingbird's. *Please, please, please taste good*. I was a little worried that between the flour and the oil, it might taste like coconut, and ironically, I had never been a fan. But if this was even close to the real thing . . . I hedged, breaking just a piece off the edge and popping it into my mouth.

It had an amazing texture—light, airy, a little spongy, but not the least bit sodden or greasy—and not a hint of coconut flavoring. Just good, old-fashioned bread!

This is it! This is exactly what I've been missing!

"Babe, this is perfect!" Ryan said after trying the piece I'd handed him. "You did it!"

"Let's see how it tastes toasted!" I squealed, cutting another slice. I had been craving a simple piece of jam-covered toast for ages. I dropped the slice into our toaster, and when it popped back up, it was nice and crispy. *And no coconut smell*, I quietly rejoiced. Grabbing a butter knife out of the drawer, I slathered the slice with some home-made strawberry jam I'd cooked a few weeks before for Asher and took a big bite. *Perfect!*

It's hard to explain what it feels like when you think you will never again experience the taste and texture of something you've always loved—even something as simple as fresh jam on toasted white bread—only to realize that you were wrong! It's one of the greatest feelings in the whole world.

I made three more loaves that week, and Ryan and I feasted on freshly grilled paninis, fried egg sandwiches, French toast—even bread pudding. There was no question about it; as far as recipes went, that simple sandwich bread was a game changer.

———————

That Saturday, as I was whipping together yet another batch, I realized that the mixture had a similar consistency to waffle batter. *Hmm, I wonder . . .*

I set aside the loaf pan, pulled out my blender, and started adding ingredients. A cup of whole cashews (I was fresh out of the expensive cashew butter from all the test loaves of bread I'd made and figured a blitz in the blender would do the same thing), a little bit of coconut oil, almond milk, eggs, some magical coconut flour, honey, baking soda, and salt. After pureeing the ingredients until they were smooth, I poured the batter into the waffle iron I never thought I'd get to use again and closed the lid.

The machine's red light went on, and steam started to escape between the two metal plates as the batter cooked. After about a minute, the two plates slowly started to lift apart, and I could see the waffles expanding. *Yes! They're rising!*

As soon as the light turned green, I took the first square out of the iron and broke off a little piece. It was gently sweet, fluffy in the center, and just a little crispy on the outside. *A little heavier and denser than a traditional waffle*, I mused, *but definitely a waffle!*

I felt almost giddy. Saturday mornings were banana chocolate pancake mornings for Ryan and me all through college, and that had become our family of three's weekend tradition as well. As much as we loved it, I had been dying to introduce Asher to waffles—the crispy outside and soft, chewy inside; the little grid of squares cradling pools of sweet maple syrup and melted butter. But I never could figure out a recipe. *This might just be it!*

I baked up two more waffles, placed them on a plate, covered them with blueberries and pure, organic maple syrup, and set them down in front of Ryan.

Immediately to Ryan's left, Asher was sitting in his high chair eyeing his plate. One of his favorite things to do was to line up all his blueberries on his tray and pretend to count them. "One, two, six, ten, mimeteen!"

"Wait!" I stopped Ryan before the fork could go into his mouth, reached back and grabbed a handful of blueberries out of the container, and set them in front of Asher along with a small piece of the original waffle. "Might as well get both my guys' opinions," I said, biting my lower lip in anticipation.

Ryan took a bite, then slowly chewed.

Well? I thought, practically climbing out of my own skin. *Say something!*

He looked over at me, and a slow smile formed on his face. "These really do taste like waffles."

"Really? You think?"

He shook his head in amazement. "They're the closest to the real deal of anything you've ever made!"

I leaned forward and threw my arms around Ryan in a hug. Over his shoulder I could see Asher chewing. All of his little blueberries were lined up in a row, but his waffle was gone!

My heart absolutely leapt with excitement.

"You did it, Dan," Ryan said, gently rocking me back and forth. "You really did it."

By now the tears were flowing. I really *had* done it. We weren't just eating healthy; we were eating well. My mind raced back to the first time I perused that list of "can't haves" on the Paleo website and honestly wondered, *What's left?* As it turns out—*everything*. If I just focused on all the things I *could* eat—meats, chicken, fish, berries, nuts, seeds, vegetables—and used my imagination to turn those humble, real-food ingredients into something fantastic, this might actually work as a "forever lifestyle" for me, as opposed to yet another short-term diet that would quickly lose its luster and fizzle out. If I could make this work, I could have it all. I could eat well *and* feel great.

11

A smile swept across my face as I read the comments below the chicken tikka masala recipe I'd posted the night before:

> This looks sooo good! —Leisa S

> I hope you're planning to bring us some leftovers! —Cindi N

There they were. My three biggest fans—my sister, my mom, and right underneath them ...

> That looks so yummy, Danielle. Need a taste tester?
> Love, Grandma Marge —Marge N

I couldn't help but laugh. No matter how many times I told Grandma that she didn't have to sign her name—that the app would automatically tell me who it was from—my grandma still signed every comment "Grandma Marge."

"Sorry, Mom," I typed. "No leftovers this time. Ryan ate the whole thing!!!!"

Leisa was right, though. It *did* look good. *That new camera really does make a difference*, I mused, eyeing the photos. In addition to the final plated shot, I had recently started adding pictures of the dish "in progress" to show the different steps. I had seen a handful of other food bloggers do it, and I liked the effect. *In fact*, I pondered, scrolling back through some of the earlier posts I'd done just using my phone, *it probably wouldn't hurt to reshoot some of these. Like this one*, I thought, looking at the poorly lit plate of grain-free lasagna. As I scrutinized the grainy, slightly sepia-toned image, my eyes inadvertently drifted down to the comment section.

> This was amazing! I couldn't believe I was not eating real lasagna noodles. I didn't even miss the meat. —Gayle

Gayle? I thought. *Who's . . . ? Wait.* My eyes widened. *I don't know this person!* I quickly scrolled down to some of the other posts I hadn't looked at for a while:

> Your recipes are impossibly good! I just can't believe how you make Paleo dishes taste so non-Paleo! —Jenn

> Made your banana chocolate chip muffins yesterday. My husband was superimpressed! Loved them! —Kimberly

> Absolutely delicious. I LOVED it and my NON SCD husband thought it was delicious too! Thank you for a wonderful recipe! —Alice

"Ryan!" I shouted.

Almost instantly, he appeared in the doorway, a panicked look on his face. "What?"

"People are reading my blog!" I said, beaming. His whole body went limp as he exhaled. "For the love, Danielle. You scared me half to death."

"I'm sorry… but look!" I shifted the screen so he could see it. "People I've never even met are reading my blog! And they like my recipes!"

"Of course they do," he said, kissing the top of my head while leaning in for a closer look. "Your food is fantastic."

My heart was practically pounding out of my chest. It was one thing to have my own family tell me they liked my food, but complete strangers? And they weren't just commenting on the pictures—they had *actually made* the recipes!

"How did they even find me?" I wondered aloud.

"Probably the same way you found your first few recipes," Ryan said, shrugging. My mind drifted back to that little forum I stumbled across back when I was first diagnosed and frantically searching for *anything* that might help. *I was so desperate back then. And scared.* I scrolled down a little further.

I just made these for Valentine's Day yesterday and they came out GREAT! Fluffy and mushroom capped like "regular" cupcakes. My last SCD baking adventure wasn't so successful. Thanks for posting! —Renee

I just made these cookies today. Per my 17-year-old, they taste "amaaaazing!" I agree <3 Thank you for the recipe. I will be adding this to my SCD collection! —Nancy

I just made these muffins tonight! They are AMAZING!!! My daughter said . . . Best. Muffin. Ever! I compromised on the

chocolate chips as I cannot tolerate chocolate, but the rest of
the family can. So I just used them in the streusel topping. I
could not believe how much they rose—the highest muffins
I have ever made . . . ! And the thing I love most about these
muffins, no tummy aches or headaches! Thank you! Thank
you! Thank you! —Kellie

"Wow," Ryan exhaled. "You've got a real following here."

"I know. Can you believe it?" I shook my head, continuing to scroll
back through my earlier posts.

My six-year-old son can't have almond flour because of a nut
allergy. Any suggestions? —Stephanie

"Gosh, they're asking questions too." I sighed.

"Hmm." Ryan stood back up and began gently massaging my
shoulders. "*Do* you have any suggestions?"

"Not really," I sat back in my chair, feeling more than slightly overwhelmed.

"Well, if anyone can figure something out," he kissed the top of
my head again, "it's you. I'm really proud of you, babe."

I reached up and grasped his hand, still resting on my shoulder. It
was pretty amazing. To think . . . all these people were actually coming to *me* for help. It was incredibly humbling. Who would have ever
guessed a plate of runny cauliflower could lead to this?

I read back over the comments. Many of them referenced their
own health issues—IBS, celiac, multiple sclerosis, lupus, diabetes. If
Ryan was right and they'd found my blog by googling their condition plus "food," that meant I wasn't the only one who believed that
changing the way you eat could have an impact on your health.

And why shouldn't they believe that? My symptoms had almost
completely vanished, I reasoned, and I had no doubt it was because of

the way I'd been eating. My only regret was that I had wasted so much time feeling miserable and dealing with all the debilitating side effects of the steroids my doctors insisted were the *only* possible solution.

I wonder how many of these poor people are dealing with the same thing, I lamented, touching the screen. *Frustrated, sick, miserable . . . alone.* Ever since this whole nightmare started, all I wanted was to feel like myself again, to live a normal life, to enjoy holidays and social gatherings with my family and friends—to be happy. To be healthy.

Well, I thought, snapping myself back to reality, *I'm not alone anymore.* And I didn't want anyone else to have to go through what I had. The medical community might not believe in the healing power of food, but I did! And not just healthy food, but delicious, flavorful, "I'd like a second helping" food.

I glanced at Stephanie's question about her son's nut allergy. I smiled. *I may not have a solution right now, but I will! And I promise you, Stephanie, whatever it is, it will be delicious!*

Over the next several weeks, the comments continued to pour in as more people started linking to AgainstAllGrain.com, discovered the blog, and reposted their favorite recipes of mine on their own sites. Then on May 21, 2012, the floodgates opened.

As I was about to post my bread recipe, I thought, *Hmm . . . plain white bread. It may not be superexciting, but it's a game-changer for me.* I was sure someone out there must be missing it as much as I did. After opting for the slightly more enticing title of "Grain-Free Sandwich Bread," I posted pictures of thick, crusty slices smothered in homemade blueberry preserves and hit Publish. The comments started coming in instantly.

You are a genius! I will bake this bread for my grandson who has type 1 diabetes (with stevia instead of honey). —Gwen

THANK YOU!! I've been missing bread so much! I can't wait to revisit some of my old favorites. Grilled cheese, here I come! So glad I found this website! —Grace

You are my hero! My little boys who are on SCD are eating nice warm bread for the first time in over a year! Thank you! —Beth

One of my clients turned me on to your website. She just brought me a slice of your sandwich bread this morning and it was to die for! By far, best Paleo bread I've ever put in my mouth! Thanks so much for the inspiration! —Brianne

By the end of the week, the recipe had been "liked" more than six hundred times, shared more than one hundred times, and had garnered more than four hundred comments—all of them positive, with the exception of a handful of people complaining about the cleanup. Because all the ingredients had to be mixed separately, it did use up a lot of bowls. But I figured the fact that it had no grains or gluten and didn't require any kneading, rising, proofing, or flour-covered countertops made up for that. Regardless, the bread was a hit, and before I knew it, the little blog that used to be no more than a place for my immediate family to touch base was getting the attention of thousands of people looking to improve their health with food.

"I've got to tell you, Dan," Ryan said, scrolling through the comments section, "it is going to be really hard to top that bread." He turned and looked at me. "What are you going to do next?"

I'd been thinking about that. As popular as the main dishes and sides were, the most effusive comments seemed to show up on the baked goods posts. Since it was virtually impossible to find a bakery item without flour, sugar, and dairy, most people who followed gluten-free, SCD, or Paleo lifestyles—me included—just assumed those foods were out of their lives forever. I couldn't speak for my readers, but I sure as heck knew what I'd been missing—chocolate chip cookies. And as Asher neared two, I realized how much I'd loved baking with my mom growing up. I wanted to be able to enjoy that pastime with him.

I had tried a bunch of recipes, but much like those first few loaves of bread, none of them tasted like chocolate chip cookies—at least not the ones *I* remembered.

I'd also done a lot of reading about what makes some cookies flat and crispy and others more cakelike, and I found Alton Brown's explanations and recipes to be the most helpful. He even had different recipes for "chewy" and "flat" cookies. (It basically boils down to which sugars and fats you use and whether the ingredients are cold or room temperature.) Me? I wanted something slightly cakey but with just a bit of chew, like the classic Nestlé Toll House cookies my mom used to bake when I was little.

My previous batches had always tasted too gritty and oily, which made me wonder if, once again, almond flour was the culprit. *Coconut flour solved the oily problem before*, I reasoned. *Might as well try it here as well.*

To combat the graininess, I decided to make the dough in my food processor to grind down the somewhat coarse almond flour even further.

Next up were the sweeteners. The recipe on the back of the chocolate chip bag called for both brown and white sugars, so I knew I also wanted to add two different sweeteners for complexity and depth of flavor. Up to this point, I had mostly been using honey because it was the only sweetener SCD considered "legal." But I knew that wouldn't give me the deep, rich, brown sugary taste I was going for. I glanced in my pantry. *I wonder if this would work*, I mused, reaching for the bag of coconut sugar I had bought the other day. I didn't have a particular recipe in mind when I tossed it into my cart. I didn't even know if my system would tolerate it. It was relatively new to the market, and I hadn't seen much info about it online, other than it had a low glycemic index and was considered Paleo-friendly. But it said *coconut*, and I knew I could eat that.

I turned the bag over in my hand and looked at the small brown crystals visible through the packaging. *It looks like brown sugar. I guess I can try adding it and see how both the cookies and my body react.*

What else? I thought, tossing the sugar onto the counter. *Ahhh . . . fat!* Almost every SCD recipe I'd seen used coconut oil, but I wasn't a big fan. It made everything taste tropical, and it melted so quickly that everything spread like crazy in the oven. Almost all of the baked goods I'd tried using it in came out dense and greasy. *Maybe this stuff would work as a substitute*, I thought, reaching for a container of palm shortening that a small family-owned business from the Philippines had sent me as a sample a few weeks before. According to the label, it had a higher melting point than coconut oil. *If it doesn't melt as fast, I might get a lighter, fluffier cookie . . . sold*, I thought, setting it down next to the coconut sugar.

I spent the next several hours experimenting with different amounts and combinations of ingredients. Every change was in small doses—a teaspoon here, a half teaspoon there. I made note of every change in different columns in my recipe journal—V1 | V2 | V3 | V4—with lines dividing them and the same ingredients in a bullet list but with notations of the small differences between them. Version 1 had one tablespoon of honey. Not sweet enough. Version 2 had two tablespoons. But they were still too greasy, so I increased the one tablespoon of coconut flour from that version to two for version 3.

Finally, after several days and about a dozen attempts, I pulled a batch of what—for all intents and purposes—appeared to be perfect Toll House cookies out of the oven.

After they had cooled for a few minutes, I tentatively picked one up and looked at it more closely. *Color looks right. Nice and cakey. No grease on the bottom.* Then I took a sniff. It smelled delicious. My mouth even started to water a little—an impressive feat, considering how many bad batches I'd taste-tested over the past week. I glanced over at Asher, who was watching me from the comfort of his high chair, fresh blueberry juice cloaking the bottom half of his face. I gave him another handful of berries so he could line them up in a row and pretend to count them. While he was occupied, I threw another batch together and got them into the oven.

Then I picked up a baked cookie again. "Here goes nothing, Ash!" I said, taking a bite.

Oh, wow . . . these are really good.

Just then, the front door opened. "Dan? You home?"

I quickly checked my watch: 5:30. Shoot. I had completely lost track of time—again. "In the kitchen!" I called out, grabbing a clean dish towel and wiping the blueberry stains off Asher's mouth.

"Hey, babe." Ryan smiled. "Wow, something smells great in here. What's for dinner?"

I looked down at Asher and laughed. "Chocolate chip cookies."

Fortunately, Ryan loved the cookies as much as I did. Nothing lacking. No detection of the "free froms." But would they pass the kid test?

Earlier that spring, Ryan and I had started having some high school and college kids from our church over for Bible study and dinner. Not only did we love the community it created around our table, it gave me a chance to test some of my new recipes. Since practically everything I made took several attempts to get "just right," we almost always had extras lying around. I'd yet to meet the college student who would turn down anything homemade—even if it wasn't four-star dining (or in some cases, two-star). That week, shortly before the group was scheduled to arrive, I whipped up a fresh batch of cookies.

Let's see their reaction to these, I thought as I placed the cookies on a serving plate. They were all far too polite to tell me if something tasted off, but expressions don't lie. If they didn't make any weird faces after biting into them, I would know I'd hit gold.

As soon as I set the plate down, the boys grabbed the cookies and devoured them. I stood off to the side, holding my breath.

Nobody said a word.

"Did you guys like the cookies?" I finally asked.

They all nodded enthusiastically, and a chorus of "Yeah!" and "They were really good" filled the air.

"They taste like the Toll House cookies my mom used to make," one of them added.

BINGO!

As soon as the boys left, I went straight to my laptop and uploaded the photos of the freshly plated cookies I'd taken earlier that day, with Asher attached to my leg. I called them Real-Deal Chocolate-Chip Cookies, and the response was almost as overwhelmingly positive as the bread recipe. Within a matter of days, the recipe had been liked and shared ten times more than even the bread recipe.

That made me realize something: *If the bread and cookies are this wildly popular, especially compared to my dinner recipes, it must be comfort foods people are looking for. Things from their past. Things they felt they lost for good when they gave up grains and dairy.*

Almost instantly, the comfort foods I'd sworn off resurfaced in my head: beef tacos, strawberry shortcake, cheese crackers, ice cream, smoothies, chicken and dumplings, berry cobbler, even pizza and doughnuts. Could I recreate each of those, too? Or at least parts of them?

Over the next few months, I continued to experiment with some of my favorite foods—cinnamon-raisin coffee cake, jam-filled cereal breakfast bars, seven-layer bars, black-bottom banana cream pie, rosemary breadsticks, pear berry crisp, French vanilla ice cream, and crispy sweet potato fries—one by one—posting my successes on the blog. Soon the requests started pouring in.

> I miss French vanilla creamer in my morning cup of coffee. Can you come up with a dairy-free version?

> I loved your dairy-free vanilla ice cream. Can you do a mint chip one?

> I really miss macaroni and cheese. Could you please create a gluten- and dairy-free version?

"Hmm . . ." I frowned at the screen.

"What's wrong?" Ryan looked up from his book at the other end of the couch.

"I got another request for mac and cheese."

"Wow," he said. "That makes like . . ."

"A lot," I said dejectedly. "I just can't seem to nail that one."

"Don't worry. You will." He winked at me and went back to his book.

I continued to scowl at the screen. With a heavy sigh, I wondered, *Why can't I figure that one out?*

"Dan," Ryan said, looking up at me. "Stop beating yourself up. It's one recipe. Look at all the people you've helped." He gestured toward the laptop.

He was right. As discouraged as I was over not being able to come up with a mac and cheese recipe (free of actual mac and cheese) to rival the creamy, golden, delectable lunchtime favorite, I couldn't help but be blown away by all the comments from readers whose lives had been changed because of the recipes I *had* managed to crack. It wasn't just other UC sufferers who contacted me, but also those living with other autoimmune diseases—multiple sclerosis, lupus, rheumatoid arthritis. I had even heard from people who found relief from autism, Lyme disease, chronic pain, and migraines. There seemed to be no limit to the healing power of food!

Desperately in need of a good virtual pep talk, I scrolled back through a few of my favorite comments.

My daughter, Amy, was diagnosed with Crohn's disease at eight years old. She struggled for years to gain weight and was on an NG feeding tube for four years until, quite by accident, someone told us about the SCD diet. At first, we were both in tears trying to make anything that tasted good, especially baked goods. So many attempts went into the trash. Then Amy stumbled upon your website. We have yet to try one recipe that doesn't taste good! In the past year and a half since finding your recipes, Amy, now nineteen, has gained eleven pounds, and her inflammation markers are normal for the first time since age eight. Most importantly, she has hope for a life that is not ruled by Crohn's disease. —Jill

I suffer from chronic Lyme and was really suffering with the treatment protocol. Once I switched my diet, the treatment started to work. When a friend introduced me to your blog, I made your chocolate cream pie and started to cry. Finally— something that tasted good and was nourishing as well. I passed congenital Lyme to my son in utero, so you can imagine my mama's guilt. This food lifestyle has not only helped him heal, but has made him feel like a normal kid again with yummy food that doesn't "hurt" him. —Sarah

My symptoms were very late MS and early ALS. I was looking at wheelchairs, because I would soon be housebound. The only treatment I knew at that time was antibiotics, which led to leaky gut and candida issues. After lots of research, I decided to take the natural route to heal my body. You were the first author/cook I stumbled upon, and after three years of natural healing, I'm now 95 percent better, working more than forty hours a week and working out four to five days a week. I have a new shot at life! —Jess

You literally saved my life. When I was forty-three, I became very sick. I spent three years trying to figure out why, and when the solution was dietary change, I did not know what to do. You taught me there was another way, and all my illness disappeared. I feel better now at fifty-two than I have in years! Thank you for your tireless recipe development, support, sharing, and kind words. Words cannot express how much your work has meant to my life. —Marco

"Now what's wrong? Did someone leave a mean comment?" Ryan said, putting down his book and walking toward me with a concerned look on his face.

"No! Not at all. It's nothing," I sniffed, the tears flowing freely. "I just . . ." I honestly couldn't even find the words. "All these people . . . All those years, I just felt so alone. And now . . ."

Ryan smiled. "You've got a whole community."

I was so, so grateful. A little in shock and disbelief, but grateful. But there was also this sense of weight on my shoulders. I had such an urgency to tell anyone who would listen that food could help. I was publishing three to five new recipes a week, yet it seemed I couldn't post them quickly enough. And it was starting to cost a lot of money to test and develop the recipes and occasionally pay someone to watch Asher so I could concentrate on taking photos and review the backlog of comments.

I also felt a bit overwhelmed. I wanted to help everyone. The log of comments waiting for answers was a little intimidating. And the requests for ingredient substitutions and cries for help in long emails in which people shared their health stories weighed heavily on me at times.

I nodded and wiped my cheeks with my sleeve. I looked at all the shares and commenters asking permission to link to my blog. "I just wish there was a way to reach more people. The blog is great, and it's definitely working. It just feels so . . . I don't know . . . hit or miss, you know? Either people find it or they don't. And I'm worried that I'm spending too much of our savings to keep up at this rate."

"So . . . ," Ryan hedged, "what are you thinking?"

I shook my head. "I don't know. Maybe an ebook?"

Ryan gave my hand a quick squeeze. "You'll think of something. You always do."

As it turned out, this time I didn't have to. Someone else came up with it for me. The email showed up in my inbox in July 2012:

> Dear Danielle,
>
> I've been following your blog, *Against All Grain*, for some time now and our family has been enjoying a number of your recipes! In fact, we had your vanilla granola as "breakfast for dinner" tonight. Thank you for all the work you put into your blog!

The writer then explained that her daughter had been diagnosed with a rare genetic condition at age six. As a consequence, they had to strictly limit the amount of sugar she ate. Her family began to follow a Paleo diet, which made a big difference.

> I have spent a lot of time doing internet research for information and new and tasty recipes to try. . . . I shared

your site with our publisher, and he thought it was fabulous! He asked me to reach out to you to see if you might be interested in writing a cookbook for us. I do hope this is something that you would consider doing, as your recipes and photos are outstanding. . . .

I look forward to hearing from you.

A publisher wants to publish a cookbook by me? I couldn't quite wrap my head around it. *Why would anyone want to publish a cookbook with me?* I wasn't a professional chef. I'd never even taken a cooking class. I wasn't on television. I was just a young mom who wanted to live a healthy life with UC without having to depend on medication and steroids.

I reread the email. *She likes the photos.* For the briefest of moments, I actually considered the idea. *Maybe I could.*

No. I'd been watching Food Network religiously, and I had loads of cookbooks and subscriptions to all the food magazines. Only "real" chefs—the kind who own restaurants and have their own TV shows—write cookbooks.

It's not like I'm Julia Child or Rachael Ray, I silently scoffed. *I'm just Danielle Walker.*

PART 3

Live Well

12

Just keep an open mind. I recalled Ryan's final words to me as he headed off to work that morning. For some reason, the whole cookbook idea made much more sense to him than it did to me.

"What could it hurt to at least call them?" he had asked. "After all, they reached out to you. They must think you can do it."

"Okay," I finally conceded. "I'll call first thing tomorrow."

Now as I held the phone in my hand, the number already entered, I was having second thoughts. *What if she was just being polite? Worse yet, what if she asks where I trained? Then what am I supposed to say? My kitchen?* I was just about to put my phone away when I remembered, *I promised Ryan I would call. He's going to ask me what happened. Shoot.* I quickly hit the call button before I could talk myself out of it. It started ringing. *They'll probably realize they made a mistake and politely rescind their offer,* I thought, pacing nervously across the living room.

"Hi, is this Kathleen?" I asked as soon as a woman's voice came on the other end.

"Yes." She sounded hesitant. I froze for a second.

"My name is Danielle Walker—" Before I could even explain why I was calling, she broke in.

"Oh, hi! I'm so glad you called!"

Really?

"First, let me tell you again why I love your recipes so much."

Huh, she really is using my recipes, I thought sitting down on the edge of the couch. *That's kind of cool.*

"As you may remember from my email, my daughter has a rare genetic condition, and I've had her on a grain-free diet to help manage it," she explained. "Every Wednesday is cereal day at her school. All the kids bring in their sugary cereals, but my little girl can't eat those. She has always felt so left out."

Poor kid. It's hard enough feeling like an outsider as an adult. I couldn't imagine dealing with it at that age.

"So," she continued, "I started looking for something that she *could* eat. I found your granola recipe online, and she loves it! So now every Wednesday I send her to school with her granola cereal and almond milk. She finally feels normal again—just like the other kids."

My eyes welled with tears as I mentally put Asher in her child's place. I would do anything for him to feel healthy. And to feel normal.

"Anyway, I showed your blog to my boss, and he suggested I reach out to see if you'd be interested in doing a cookbook with us."

The line went quiet. *Say something.*

"How exactly would that work?" I asked, hoping I sounded more confident and professional than I felt.

As she started describing the process, I quickly grabbed one of Ryan's empty legal pads and frantically scribbled down notes.

"Who does your photos on your blog?" she asked.

"I do." I cringed a little. So much for sounding like a professional.

"Well, then," she said enthusiastically, "we'd love for you to do all the food photos too."

I wasn't sure I heard her correctly. "Are you sure?" I asked. "I'm not a trained photographer or anything. My pictures are okay, but . . . for a book?" *Wait.* I caught myself. *Am I really thinking about doing this?*

"We *love* what you've done so far with the photos," she assured me. "Of course, we could also work with you to arrange for a photographer to take photos of you in your kitchen."

"Okay. Thanks," I said. "Is there a theme or anything in particular you would want me to focus on?"

"You can come up with the theme and pick anything you want to write about. But we are finding Paleo recipes like yours to be popular right now," she replied.

Anything? I wouldn't even know where to start.

We talked for a few more minutes. It all sounded so lovely and hypothetical. And then . . .

"Tell you what," Kathleen said. "Why don't I go ahead and send you a contract outlining all of this."

"Oh, okay." I said. "That would be great. Thanks." *Is this really how it works?* I promised Kathleen I would call if I had any questions about the contract, and we said our goodbyes. I clicked the End Call button and sat on the couch speechless. I looked over at Asher, who had been playing with his fleet of die-cast Pixar cars all lined up on the floor a few feet away.

"Well, Ash," I said, dumfounded, "it looks like your mommy is going to write a book."

A few days later, the contract arrived via email. Ryan, now officially a licensed attorney, agreed to look it over for me. The only details I took note of were the number of recipes and photos they were asking for—"a minimum of 120"—and the due date—"six months from signing."

"Do you have 120 recipes?" Ryan asked.

"Well . . ." I quickly counted in my head. "No." I did have several dozen on the blog, but Kathleen wanted me to come up with mostly new recipes so the people following me there would have a reason to buy the book. That made sense to me. And book or no book, I was committed to posting two new recipes a week. Once I did the math, I realized that between a cookbook and my blog, I would have to come up with about 140 new recipes—in six months!

Aside from the question of how I was actually going to do it, Ryan thought the contract looked good. In a naive whirlwind of excitement, I signed it and sent it back to Kathleen. The expense of developing dozens of new recipes through trial and error in such a short period of time never even occurred to me. Nor did the added challenge of pulling together and photographing a 350-plus page cookbook while caring for a toddler who was becoming more active every day. *I'm going to need a ton of ingredients, and probably a babysitter to watch Asher a couple of days a week.* My mind started reeling. *This is going to cost us a fortune.*

I took a deep breath to get my bearings. Then I panicked.

"I need to take a photography class," I told Ryan. "I can't shoot an entire cookbook the way I'm doing the blog. I don't even know what I'm doing!"

I sometimes took up to two hundred photos of the same dish (and unlike people, food doesn't move!) before I saw one I liked. I never could seem to figure out what I'd done right with the lighting or angle to replicate it, and my photo sessions would often end with me throwing my hands up and saying I was going to quit the whole thing.

When I first started using the Canon Rebel Ryan gave me for Christmas, it was not unusual for him to have to wait forty-five minutes for dinner while I fumbled with it, trying to create an appetizing photo before allowing anyone to eat the food. By the time we sat down to eat, everything was cold. Ryan was such a trouper, but I could tell he was somewhat annoyed! After a few months of carrying on like that at every meal, I decided that testing and photographing new recipes during Asher's nap time was my best option. I could reheat everything at dinnertime so they wouldn't have to watch their food turn cold and gray.

Even so, Ryan was a little concerned about the expense of a professional photography course—especially given how much I had already spent stocking and restocking our pantry, not to mention the medical bills we were paying off in installments every month. All told, my condition was costing us a small fortune. I was starting to see why they worked "for richer, for poorer, in sickness and in health" into wedding vows.

While we both agreed that a full course in photography was definitely *not* in our budget or the time allotted for the book, I was able to convince Ryan to let me sign up for a one-day intensive food photography class.

I had a blast learning about the different lenses, scenery settings, and ways to use light to make even the simplest dishes look their very best. I was also stunned at how much I didn't know. I walked into that class thinking I would have the best camera there. Instead, mine looked like a child's toy compared to the machines the other students had. And I was shell-shocked to see that most of the beautiful surfaces under the dishes I longingly looked at in food magazines and websites were fake rectangular surfaces painted to look like countertops or reclaimed wood tables. I always figured these people just had really cool furniture they were using!

In the class, I also learned so many new terms: *f-stops, bounce cards, depth of focus, remote shutters, tripods.* I had never heard of any of them. Before that class, whenever I set up to take a shot, I would hunch over the food with my camera in hand, one foot perched precariously on a table, the other balancing a white cardboard piece between my toes for reflection. My other hand, Twister style, snapped the photo on the computer. *Right foot, blue!*

I already felt insecure about writing a cookbook because I wasn't a trained chef; now I felt anxious about not being a professional photographer. But Kathleen and her boss seemed to believe in me, and I didn't want to let them down.

After the class was over, I approached Ryan with yet another request.

"I really need a better camera."

"How much better?" he asked.

"Well . . . ," I hedged. My Rebel was good enough for the blog, but everyone else in the class had high-end professional models with what seemed like a dozen different lenses and many special features, and they swore those extras made all the difference. "I asked the instructor what she would recommend for someone like me, and she suggested this camera"—I handed Ryan the printout the instructor had given me—"with this lens. She said if she could only start with one lens, it would be that one," I said.

He let out his standard chirp of a chortle, which he always did when a price looked ridiculous.

I could almost see his brain reviewing our most recent bank statement as I spoke.

"I know it's a lot," I told him. "It's just that, well . . . if I'm going to do this, I want to it right."

Ryan stood up from the table and let out a long breath. Then he shook his head, laughed, and said, "Okay, but at that price, this is the *only* lens you're going to start with."

"Thank you!" I squealed and threw my arms around his neck.

"You're welcome," he said, hugging me back. "It's less expensive than a hospital bill."

My fancy new camera in hand, it was time to get started. I was adamant that the cookbook be a mesh of healthy, gluten-free, GAPS,

SCD, and Paleo recipes. Based on the comments and feedback I had been receiving on Facebook, I knew the odds were that people struggling with autoimmune diseases would try some, if not all of those diets, and I wanted my book to have something for everyone.

The following months were a nonstop flurry of grocery store runs, late nights tinkering in the kitchen, countless hours analyzing my recipe journals, and entire afternoons styling, staging, and snapping photos. And washing dishes. So many dishes.

The phrase "Here, try this" took the place of "Good morning" or "How was your day?" whenever Ryan walked into the kitchen. By the time 2013 rolled around, my family and Ryan's coworkers had sampled close to 120 soups, salads, main courses, desserts, smoothies, and snacks. When people saw me coming, they didn't know whether to turn and run the other way or grab a fork and surrender. Their feedback, however, was invaluable: "It's a little salty." "I'm not sure I like the texture." "Is it supposed to be this dense?" I even went back and tweaked some of the recipes that had been on my blog for over a year. Then late one evening . . .

"Ryan?"

"What's wrong?" he asked groggily, not lifting his head from the pillow. "Is it Asher?"

"No . . . look," I said, tilting my laptop in his direction.

He glanced up, his eyes squinting to adjust to the light from the lamp on my nightstand. "Dan," he moaned, "you promised not to bring that thing to bed with you."

"I know, but look!" I pressed. "It's finished."

He lifted his head. "Really?"

"I think so," I said scrolling through the pages. "I mean, it still needs to be designed and everything, but I think this is it." I didn't know whether to smile or cry. I opted for both. I had actually done it. Over a hundred recipes—from dairy-free clam chowder to zucchini bread—each complete with a full ingredients list, step-by-step directions, tips, tricks, tidbits, and of course, a stunning close-up photograph.

"You know," Ryan said, sitting up for a closer look, "that fancy camera lens really did make a huge difference."

"Worth every penny." I smiled through tears.

First thing the next morning, I uploaded the colossal file to Kathleen's Dropbox—a full month and a half *before* my deadline. While enjoying two of my new favorite recipes, an asparagus, leek, and prosciutto quiche and a fresh-brewed chai latte, I calculated the final number of recipes in my head: 163. I'd created several more than the contract asked for, but this was my one and only book. I'd wanted to put everything in it I could think of, and I had.

Five months later, after countless hours of working with the editor and realizing I didn't truly know how to write a recipe, a package arrived at our door. As soon as I picked it up, I knew. I didn't have to look at the return address—the size, shape, and weight were dead giveaways. Plus it was roughly a month before the book's July 30, 2013, release date.

"Ryan," I called out excitedly. "It's here! It's finally here!"

By the time Ryan arrived on the front step, Asher clinging to his legs, I was crying like a baby.

"Hold on," he said, digging his phone out of his back pocket. "I want to record this."

My hands were shaking as I tore the padded envelope open. I looked inside. The book was even thicker than I'd expected. I gently pulled it out of the envelope and watched as the front cover slowly came into focus in front of me: *Against All Grain: Delectable Paleo Recipes to Eat Well and Feel Great.* There I was, smiling back at myself, a partially sliced loaf of my sandwich bread and a heaping dish of Greek gyro pasta with lamb meatballs proudly displayed on the table in front of me. I ran my fingers over the words "Written and photographed by Danielle Walker," my heart bursting with joy.

"That's you, Mama!" Asher said, pointing at my picture on the cover.

"That's me!" I nodded and smiled back at him through tears. "Mommy made a book."

"Great job, Mommy," Ryan smiled from behind his phone, using the special voice he always used when talking to Asher.

"Do you want to see you?" I asked, pulling Asher onto my lap on the bottom step of the entryway. He nodded enthusiastically.

Ryan moved behind me and started recording over my shoulder as I flipped through the colorful pages, stopping every time I got to a picture that featured Asher helping me in the kitchen.

"Who's that?" I asked him.

"Me!" he happily chirped back, touching the image.

I was somewhere between disbelief and euphoria as I looked through the pages and saw how it had come together. All my long days and late nights had paid off. I had designed every page, selecting the font choices and colors and working in a pretty watercolor splash on almost every page. Even though it was a cookbook, I wanted it to feel whimsical, personal, and pretty—something people would want to keep out on a coffee table. Something to show that healthy food didn't have to look drab and boring. It was almost like flipping through a family album—I'd recreated so many of the recipes from longtime family favorites. Virtually every page brought back a flood of childhood memories. *Just like great food should*, I thought.

After I had leafed through the entire book, I went back to the introduction. I had written and rewritten it so many times I could have recited it by heart. Next to it was a full-page photo of Ryan, Asher, and me smiling in front of a plate of chocolate cupcakes frosted with swirls of Italian meringue. I had seen the picture a month or so before when approving the final photo placements. But somehow seeing the photo of the three of us smiling in the printed book—my loving, supportive husband with his arm around me while

I cradled our little boy in my arms, and *me*, happy, healthy, *flourishing*—hit me harder than I expected.

I traced the image with my finger and thought back five years to that modest little hospital in Uganda, when I lay deathly ill, emaciated, malnourished, and terrified. I hadn't been sure what was wrong with me or even if I'd make it home alive. I looked at Asher's happy little face smiling back at me from the page and thought about the devastating loss of our twins and all the sleepless nights I'd spent asking God, *Why?* I looked at Ryan smiling down at me in the photo and thought about the countless sacrifices he'd made on my behalf.

I looked up at Ryan—Asher snuggled in my arms—my eyes brimming with tears.

"Thank you," I said, my voice cracking with emotion.

"For what?" he asked, genuinely perplexed.

I shook my head, trying and failing to find the right words. "Everything," I finally said, as tears cascaded down my cheeks.

Ryan smiled, set his phone down on the step, and sat behind me, his arms wrapped around mine, which were wrapped around Asher. The tears were flowing freely now. After five years of seemingly indescribable pain, loss, and heartache, I finally had everything I'd always wanted.

———————

As thrilling as holding that first copy and enjoying that moment with Ryan and Asher were, I was absolutely giddy about sharing the news with my Facebook and blog followers, many of whom had encouraged me along the way. The reaction was . . . not what I expected.

"Uh-oh," I said as I scrolled through the comments.

"What?" Ryan said incredulously. "Don't tell me they're not excited—"

"Actually," I said, "they're more than excited."

"So . . ." he hedged, "why the 'uh-oh'?"

"They want to meet me—in person."

"Well, that's great! Isn't it?"

It was and it wasn't. The truth is, I wanted to meet them, too. After all, we were a community—a family. Their support was the reason the book existed. And I couldn't think of a more appropriate way to say thank you than to do it face-to-face. Unfortunately, a national book tour is superexpensive, and it just wasn't in the budget.

I explained to my followers that my publisher hadn't planned a tour, and that quite honestly, Ryan and I didn't have the finances to pull it off on our own. Then I closed my laptop and went to bed, a little deflated that I couldn't fulfill their request.

The next morning after I put Asher down for his first nap, I sat down to begin responding to comments and questions on my blog and social media. I clicked the post where I had replied the night before and couldn't believe what I read: "You should set up a fundraising page! We can all contribute and get you out to the cities you want to visit."

Wow. Surely this is the only reader thinking of this, especially since we will have to charge for the cookbook. And not the $9.99 I had suggested to the publisher, but $34.95.

My eyes scrolled the comments that followed, and there it was over and over again.

"Yes! I'd be happy to help donate so I can meet you!"

"What a great idea! Please let us know if you set one up."

Over the next twenty-four hours, the number of little blue thumbs-up icons next to the comments kept climbing, indicating more and more support for this idea. I hesitated, but thought it couldn't hurt to try, so later that night, Ryan helped me set up a crowdfunding campaign on Indiegogo. I posted the link on my blog along with the following message:

I cannot express enough how thankful I am for all the support you have shown me over the past couple of years and throughout the book-writing process. I want more than anything to travel to your cities and meet all of you in person to express my gratitude, but we have virtually no budget left over after creating this book, so I need your help!

I am offsetting some of the costs by staying with friends and family when available and gathering up any and all airline miles we have, but will need help with the remaining transportation, airfare, lodging, and food budget. I am going to make the tour happen somehow regardless of [whether] this gets fully funded, but I really think this is doable!

"What's wrong?" Ryan asked after I posted the message.

"I don't know," I said. "I really do want to meet everyone, but do people really *do* this?"

Ryan looked at me thoughtfully for a second, then said, "You're only asking them to contribute $1.50, Dan. That's less than a cup of coffee."

"I suppose that's true." I sighed, looking back at the screen. Then before I could hit Refresh to see if anyone had responded, Ryan reached over and flipped my laptop shut.

"Try not to think about it," he said. "Give it till Monday. If nobody has given by then, you'll have your answer."

Well, that's a grim thought. Still, I knew he had a point. I had been open and honest with my followers from day one. I had opened up about things a lot more delicate and embarrassing than this, and they had never been anything but supportive and encouraging. Honestly, that's what I loved so much about this online community. Sometimes it's the circumstances nobody would ever choose for themselves that bind people together most.

On Monday morning, I checked the site and wept with joy. Not only was I going to meet my community, I was going to do so in eight cities nationwide.

I spent the next several days cold-calling bookstores—wherever the Pioneer Woman or the Barefoot Contessa had gone on their last tours—trying to set up signings. Most of the time, I was shot down. "It's too much work" and "It would cost too much to market the event" was the familiar refrain. The people I talked to were always polite, but in essence they were telling me that they couldn't take a chance on a never-heard-of author coming, only to have fifteen people show up.

At first, I quietly accepted that response. After all, I'm no Ina or Ree. But after the fourth or fifth time, right as they were about click off, I would blurt out, "I have twenty thousand followers on Facebook! They raised the funds for me to come see them, so I know they'll come out."

That usually made the bookstore operator pause. At the very least, it kept them from hanging up for a few extra seconds.

"You wouldn't have to do any of the legwork," I continued. "I'll promote the events. You would just need to have books on hand."

I eventually booked eight stops. It wasn't much, but I didn't care. I was just excited to get out and meet the people who had been supporting me all these years.

To be honest, when I arrived at the first few stores, I half expected to see a handful of people lingering around a card table somewhere in the back. Instead, I was stunned to see lines out the front door and wrapped around the store. Most of the booksellers ran out of books within twenty minutes, but nobody seemed to mind. They all waited patiently in line for a chance to say hello and to tell me their stories. Many were in tears, overcome with gratitude for the way *Against All Grain* had changed their health, their approach to eating, and their lives.

I watched one woman walk slowly toward my table, clearly

struggling to put one foot in front of the other. Her hair was thin and her collarbone protruded under her blouse. I knew that look, and I had a feeling I might know her story intimately.

She told me she had driven six hours with her young daughters to see me. "I've been sick for most of my daughters' lives," she explained through tears. "I've never even been able to make chocolate chip cookies with them."

Cue my tears. I thought of Asher and understood her pain. What mom doesn't dream of someday baking chocolate chip cookies with her kids, watching their little faces light up as they watch that first gooey batch come out of the oven and smell that delectable sugary-sweet aroma filling the air.

"When I started following your recipes, my health started to improve, and I was finally able to get out of bed," she continued. "And then I found your Real-Deal Chocolate-Chip Cookie recipe." Her voice cracked as she gently rubbed her daughters' backs. "Thank you so much."

Another mom asked me to sign her book to her son, who exhibited behaviors associated with autism.

"He loves your recipes," she gushed. "I couldn't get him to eat any grain- or dairy-free foods until we found your blog." Her eyes began to fill. "You're a hero in the autism community. We even have a Facebook group where we talk about your recipes."

"How is your son doing now?" I asked. Over the past several months, I had heard from moms of children on the spectrum commenting on how the diet was helping their kids manage their symptoms. Curious, I'd done a little research and discovered that many kids with autism spectrum disorder (ASD) suffer from GI issues, including leaky gut. Researchers have also discovered that the gut microbiome—the concentration of good and bad bacteria—is often out of balance in those with ASD, just like Dr. Stark explained mine was.

"He's doing beautifully!" she beamed. "Almost completely symptom-free!"

One after another, men, women, and teens approached me, sharing their stories and thanking me for helping them find a way to effectively manage their symptoms without relying on medication and without having to give up all the rich flavors, tastes, and textures of the foods they loved. Some of their spouses even commented that they had been feeling noticeably better themselves after following the diet, even though they didn't necessarily need to eat this way. That actually *didn't* surprise me. When Ryan started eating what I did, he also noticed some improvements in his sleep, moods, and digestion. And when he had wheat or dairy while at a work lunch or out with the guys, he noticed a bit of discomfort or more brain fog.

The tour was incredibly humbling and, at times, overwhelming. With the success of the first reader-funded eight stops, my publisher offered to send me to eight more on their dime, for a total of sixteen stops in two months. All the late events, early flights, emotional sharing of stories, and eating out constantly was starting to take a toll on my body. While I was still out on tour, I noticed some mild cramping and fatigue. Though the symptoms weren't severe, I was terrified—and a little angry. *Really?* I thought, *I'm supposed to go out there tonight and tell all these people about how food saved my life and now I'm sick again?*

"Danielle, don't get worked up about it," Ryan told me on the phone when I called him from my hotel in Chicago. "This is just your life. It's going to ebb and flow. These people need to hear *that*, too."

I could feel every inch of the 2,800 miles separating us at that moment.

"But I feel like such a failure," I said as I wept. "They're going to think I'm a fraud."

"No, they won't," he reassured me. "They all know the diet works. That's why they're there."

"But—"

He quickly (and wisely) cut me off. "They also get that the occasional flare-up is going to happen. Don't forget, Dan, a lot of these people are suffering with the same condition you have. They've been there. They get it. You are not a failure, babe. Or a fraud."

I knew he was right. This was just a mental block I had to get past. I just hoped my experience wouldn't discourage people from trying the recipes or buying the book.

Three weeks after *Against All Grain* released, I got my answer. I was home briefly between stops, sipping a mug of bone broth I'd whipped together the night I arrived home, when my publisher called me.

"Congratulations, Danielle! You made the *Times*."

I had no idea what he was talking about. "What does that mean?" I asked.

"The *New York Times* Best Sellers list," he said.

"Oh," I still wasn't entirely sure what that meant. "Is that . . . *good*?"

"That's the best you can get," he said, chuckling. "You're right up there with Ree, Ina, and Rachael."

Wow. While I was ecstatic to be in the company of the ladies I had looked up to and, in fact, modeled my blog and business after, I was even more excited to realize that my book being on that list meant that the way I was eating wasn't just a niche market. Tens of thousands of other people were eating this way too!

"Listen," my publisher continued. "We were just thinking . . . , how about a second book?"

I almost choked on my broth. "Another one? I literally just finished *this* one." At that moment, the thought of heading back into the kitchen with another deadline looming made my stomach churn.

He chuckled. "Just think about it. You've clearly struck a nerve here. People are loving these recipes. I'm sure they'd love even more."

As I finished up the tour, I started casually asking people what kind of recipes they'd like to see next. The overwhelming response:

"easy meals." That made sense. Even I had to admit that some of my recipes were a little time-consuming, and I had the advantage of being a stay-at-home mom with just one little guy. I could understand the challenge of finding the time to do thirty to forty minutes of prep with a full-time job and more than one child.

As it happens, I was about to find out. Shortly after telling my publisher yes, I discovered I was pregnant with our second child—due the same month as the second cookbook.

At least I know I'll have nine or more symptom-free months, I mused. *Maybe this won't be so bad after all.*

13

The room began closing in on me. I couldn't breathe. I just held Ryan's hand and stared numbly at the ultrasound monitor, willing—with every fiber of my being—for the doctor's diagnosis to be wrong. *Please, God, let it be a mistake.*

The perinatologist Dr. Veerman had referred us to solemnly shook his head. His words "severe abnormalities" and "not compatible with life" echoed in my mind.

"This isn't something either of you caused," he assured us. "It's a rare genetic mutation. I'm afraid there's nothing we can do." And just like that, all my dreams for this precious little girl, whom Ryan and I had already named Aila Jane, started shifting into a terrible nightmare.

The anguish I experienced over the next several months was far worse than anything I had ever walked through with my disease. When I lost our twins, I couldn't have imagined anything worse. I had been wrong. This was unbearable. Ryan and I spent the remainder of my pregnancy wrestling in prayer, asking for a miracle, yet bracing for the worst.

On Tuesday, June 24, 2014, the worst happened. Aila Jane was born at 7:53 p.m., weighing one pound and 5.8 ounces. We had the immense joy of knowing her on this earth for forty-six minutes before she went to be with Jesus. Her heart and lungs just weren't strong enough.

I held her for twelve hours before surrendering her to the nurses and kissing her goodbye for the final time. And as I was wheeled out of the elevator in the hospital to our waiting car, with nothing more than a memory box filled with her blankets, her tiny footprints, and her lingering scent, I wailed a guttural cry that echoed in those hospital walls and hit back on me like a freight train.

The weeks that followed were dark. I became an inconsolable wreck, barely even able to get myself out of bed. I had to sleep with the lights on so I wouldn't wake up in a terror, wondering where Aila was, or if I was still in the hospital. I checked out with heavy pain pills in an attempt to numb a different type of torment. I would sometimes leave the house for hours without telling Ryan, and without my phone, taking hikes or drives and wishing to not return. I was a ghost of a mother to Asher and farmed him out to family and friends most days so he wouldn't have to see me in that state. Tears came randomly and frequently. People reached out to offer their condolences, but I couldn't be comforted.

One day Ryan poked his head tentatively into our darkened bedroom. "Dan?" The clock on my nightstand read 9, but I honestly couldn't have told you whether it was night or day. "I know the timing of this isn't the greatest," he said, sitting down on the edge of the bed, "but your cookbook is scheduled to release in three months. Maybe we should push it back?"

I knew what he was saying. I had considered it myself. The stress of a book release—with all the travel and media, in the midst of trying to grieve—might be too much for me to handle. The last thing I needed was another full-blown flare-up. And yet part of me craved a return to normalcy—if such a thing were even possible.

"No," I said, pulling myself into a sitting position. "Aila was with me the whole time I wrote that cookbook. I want to honor her life by seeing it through."

"You're sure?" Ryan asked, taking my hand.

I took a deep breath and nodded. "I'm sure."

Honestly, I wasn't. Still, I couldn't hole away from the world forever. I began focusing all my energy on being present for Asher. He needed me. And day by day, a little more light worked its way into my life—through Asher's infectious giggle, Ryan's warm and tender hugs, our parents' loving support, and the Against All Grain community's encouragement. They filled my inbox with heartfelt messages of comfort and solidarity from those who had walked similar paths. I had made the difficult decision to share our story with my blog followers and was overwhelmed by their response. I started to think that perhaps this book tour could be the best thing for me. It could be my reentry into the "real" world and an opportunity to thank all the wonderful people who had been standing beside us through this incredibly difficult season.

Before the September release of *Meals Made Simple: Gluten-Free, Dairy-Free, and Paleo Recipes to Make Anytime*, my publisher and I began planning another book tour. We set a preliminary list of cities, some repeats such as Chicago, Houston, Atlanta, Toronto, New York, and San Diego, and some new ones, including Boston, Minneapolis, Vancouver, Seattle, Portland, and Denver. For this tour, I would bring Ryan and Asher with me to as many of the locations as I could for support. Ironically, the tour ended up being just what the doctor ordered.

Being surrounded by that community was a tremendous source

of comfort. And the number of mothers who had lost babies and came out to support our family was overwhelming. The icing on the cake? This second cookbook also hit the *New York Times* Best Sellers list.

As I began to be offered media opportunities with TV shows like *Access Hollywood* and *The Doctors* and magazines including *O*, *People*, and *Redbook*, I made sure I was completely transparent about my health. The last thing I wanted was to mislead anybody.

"You cured yourself," the interviewer would inevitably say, looking for the quick and easy sound bite.

"No," I would quickly but politely correct them, "my disease is still there. It's not gone. It will never be gone. But I *am* managing it through food and the way I eat." It might not have been as sensational or as headline-grabbing a response as they were hoping for, but it was an honest one.

Then, just as everything was starting to return to normal, I called out to my husband from our master bath.

"Ryan, it's starting again."

To be perfectly candid, neither of us was surprised. Given the intensity of the hormonal changes following Aila's birth—not to mention the crushing grief and post-traumatic stress—combined with the pressure that came from flying to a new city every day, back-to-back book signings almost every night, and 6:00 a.m. wake-up calls for television interviews, a flare-up seemed inevitable.

"It's okay," Ryan said reassuringly. "We were expecting this. Don't panic. You know what to do."

I did. I immediately started the strict elimination diet and made a big batch of SCD chicken soup and bone broth. Ryan and my mom took turns keeping an eye on Asher so I could get extra sleep. I did *not* want to have a repeat of what happened after Asher's birth.

Despite my initial concern, the soup, bone broth, and elimination diet did the trick, and within a few weeks, my symptoms had calmed down significantly. I started to feel like myself again—just in time for Christmas.

Though I didn't feel 100 percent by then, the flare-up never got out of control. I didn't lose any weight; I didn't have to go to the hospital; I didn't need a blood or iron transfusion; and I didn't have to go back on the prednisone—all thanks to food. It felt like a miracle. But it wasn't the only one. That Christmas Eve—six months to the day after we lost Aila—I gave Ryan the best present ever.

"I'm pregnant."

The fear of possibly losing another child put me into emotional overdrive. Every medical appointment brought a fresh round of anxiety. I became hypervigilant about sensing the baby's every movement. If I didn't feel enough kicks during my daily count, I drove to Dr. Veerman's office and requested a nonstress test. And I ate fully Paleo. No exceptions.

I knew my disease had absolutely nothing to do with Aila's condition or passing—Dr. Veerman reassured me of that every time I showed up at her door in a panic asking her to check the baby's heartbeat. But I still wanted to be the healthiest I possibly could be during this pregnancy to avoid any complications.

All my paranoia and anxiety aside, the pregnancy went smoothly, and on August 28, 2015, I gave birth to a healthy baby boy, whom we named Easton—for the rising of the sun, the dawning of a new day. A new page. The second they placed that chunky ten-pound bundle of joy onto my chest, my heart nearly burst.

Still, I couldn't seem to suppress the anxiety and paranoia. When we took Easton home, I was scared to death he was going to die. I didn't sleep. I was always on alert. I constantly checked his breathing to make sure he was okay. If he didn't move for more than a few minutes, I would pick him up, panicked, and gently shake him awake.

Multiple times I was convinced he was gone, and I became an emotional wreck all over again. Poor Asher seemed to have similar fears. Easton was home three full weeks before Asher asked to hold him. I think we were all a little afraid of getting too attached.

Ryan was reaching his limit. He had been my rock throughout my entire battle. He took care of me when I was sick, held me when I was frightened, and prayed with me when I needed strength. He was the one who encouraged me to start the blog that had become both my calling and my career, as well as an oasis for tens of thousands of people struggling with autoimmune diseases and food allergies. He encouraged me to eat well and stand up for myself when dealing with medical professionals. He acted as both mom and dad to Asher when I was too sick or incapacitated to be there for our son myself. He was constantly giving, constantly sacrificing, without asking anything in return. And then the one time he did . . .

"Babe," I said as Ryan headed toward the door in his running shorts and shoes, "could you stay? We need you here. *I* need you."

"Danielle." He sounded exhausted. "This is really important to me. I'm not going to be gone all day. I just need one hour to go running and clear my head and have some time for me to process everything. Just one hour."

It finally hit me. Between work, taking care of me, and helping with the kids, Ryan never got a break. Only later did I learn that for years as he was taking care of me and then caring for our newborns—which he had never done on his own before—he occasionally would sit on the stairs and cry. During all those years of being my rock, he could never crack or grieve because one of us had to be strong. Now all he wanted was an hour to himself to run and work out. To destress and refresh.

"Okay," I said apologetically. "I understand. Go." I wrapped my arms around his waist and gave him a quick hug. "You deserve some Ryan time."

As I stood in the doorway and watched him jog off, an all-too-familiar question ran through my head. *How did I ever get so lucky?* From then on I made a point to occasionally encourage Ryan to get out and take care of himself.

Once Ryan turned the corner, I went back inside and checked on the boys. Asher was quietly watching a cartoon in the living room, and three feet away, Easton was fast asleep in his crib. *Okay, back to work*, I told myself, positioning my laptop so I could see both of my sons. I was in the middle of putting together my third cookbook, *Celebrations: A Year of Gluten-Free, Dairy-Free, and Paleo Recipes for Every Occasion*.

When I scrolled through the chapters on Easter brunch and summer showers, a smile crept across my face. I was still pregnant with Easton when we shot those photos, so I was constantly trying to hide my growing bump with trays of food or flowing tops.

As usual, both Ryan and Asher were featured heavily throughout the book, and it made me happy to think that in some small way, Easton was in the book as well. After he arrived, I cooked and tested the remainder of the recipes with him strapped to my chest in a carrier—my adorable little test kitchen buddy. By this time, Asher was in school during the mornings, so it was wonderful to have that special time alone with Easton. And when we shot the last half of the book, I pulled him into as many photos as he was awake for. The pictures of him in a little lion Halloween costume, which he donned in the middle of February, and another of his big blue eyes staring at his sweet cousin Kellen in the gingerbread scene are among my favorites.

Then, just like clockwork, nine months after Easton was born and my hormones were starting to go back to their prepregnancy levels, my symptoms began to return—right in the middle of the cover shoot.

I had learned from Dr. Veerman that with the many complex

hormonal and immune-related shifts that occur during pregnancy, it is actually very common for women to be diagnosed with auto-immune diseases postpartum, especially those with a genetic pre-disposition to the condition. I did a bit of additional research on my own and discovered that four out of five diagnoses of autoimmune disease are made in women, most of whom are of reproductive age. Environmental and emotional triggers such as depression, anxiety, or feelings of being overwhelmed—all common after childbirth—can increase the chance of a flare-up. The physical stress of birthing a baby along with the sleep deprivation and nutrient defi-ciencies that follow can serve as triggers as well—not to mention the C-sections and antibiotics I'd had. For those diagnosed before pregnancy, postpartum flares are especially prevalent. I read that it is also common for mothers to develop gut permeability postpar-tum due to the use of antibiotics as well as environmental stressors.

That had definitely been *my* body's pattern.

As soon as I noticed the first symptoms emerging, I immediately started the strict elimination diet and went back on all the supple-ments Dr. Walters had prescribed back in 2011. But the inflamma-tion and pain became so bad that I was stuck back in bed. And it seemed with each flare-up, some new symptom would show itself. This one hit me right between the eyes—literally.

A few days after I began to notice symptoms, I awoke to my right eye hurting. It was so swollen I could barely open it. When I forced it open, the light burned and everything looked blurry. *It must be pink eye*, I thought. *Great, on top of the flare-up. At least it happened after we shot the cover.*

By the next day, both eyes were throbbing and barely able to open. I finally went to an ophthalmologist, who told me I had iritis, a debilitating and frightening inflammatory eye condition that can happen when the body experiences chronic inflammation during a

UC flare-up. It cleared up after treatment with steroid drops, which thankfully caused no side effects.

The other symptoms, however, kept getting worse. Over the next two weeks, I dropped twenty pounds. I was so weak that I could only come out of my room to kiss Asher goodbye before school and to nurse Easton—once in the morning and once at bedtime. All told, I think I saw my boys for a total of about forty-five minutes a day.

Because Ryan couldn't take any more time off work, we hired a wonderful nanny to care for the boys during the day, and in the evenings, our parents took turns helping out. Nearby family became invaluable.

I was so frustrated with myself. My whole mission had been to tell people they could heal themselves with food—and here I was stuck in bed with a horrendous flare-up. Sensing that I was on the verge of going into an emotional death spiral, Ryan quickly pointed out what I was too sick and discouraged to realize.

"Danielle, yes, this is a flare-up, but you know what? This is the second big flare you've experienced since Asher was born that you didn't have to go to the hospital. You didn't need a blood transfusion."

"But this flare-up is so much worse than the last one," I lamented. "I'm eating all the right things. Why does this keep happening?"

"Some people's diseases are more intense than others," he said calmly. "Plus, you just had a C-section and antibiotics, your hormones are all out of whack, you've got a newborn in the house who isn't sleeping, you just finished writing another cookbook, *and* you're still grieving the loss of Aila. Take a step back and give yourself some grace, okay?"

As usual, Ryan was right. One of the hardest things about this disease was coming to grips with the fact that it would *always* be there. Sometimes when I would go into remission for months on end, as during a pregnancy, it was easy to forget I still had it. I could keep myself healthy for months—possibly years—at a time, but at some point, the perfect storm of external factors—a virus or bug, stress, lack of sleep, hormonal shifts, antibiotics—could trigger my symptoms all over again. I would never fully beat it. But changing the way I ate was helping me manage it and—until now—keeping the flare-ups from spiraling out of control. This time around, however, the external storm was just too powerful, and my system couldn't handle it.

A few days later, my symptoms hadn't improved, so as a precaution, Ryan and I made an appointment to see Dr. York, the GI who treated me after we were fired by Dr. Benedict when Asher was still a baby.

"I'm writing you a prescription for prednisone," he said, scribbling away on his pad.

I looked at Ryan, stunned. Not so much that he was prescribing prednisone—which Ryan and I called "the devil drug" because of its effect on me. I actually expected that. It was the knee-jerk way in which he did it. *He's not even going to run a blood test first? See if anything's different? Just go straight to the devil drug?*

"Unbelievable," I said to Ryan as we walked out of his office.

He just shook his head in frustration. "Well, one thing's for sure: We're not filling that prescription," he said adamantly.

"No argument here," I agreed.

Since my body wasn't responding to the supplements and homeopathic remedies from Dr. Walters as it had before, I decided to see Dr. Hestor, a medical doctor specializing in functional medicine, to explore alternative healing therapies. Like a naturopath, I knew an MD with this specialty would focus on treating my whole person rather than simply treating my disease according to standard clinical protocol. At the same time, I valued the perspective of conventional medicine and wanted to consult a physician who took an integrative approach to discern what was going on internally. It was also comforting to know that she could write prescriptions for medications if necessary.

Dr. Hestor did a series of blood and stool tests, which revealed a small bacterial overgrowth in my intestines and, as expected, very high levels of inflammation. She prescribed additional nutritional supplements so I wouldn't become deficient in essential nutrients like potassium, as I had in the past. And to combat the dehydration and anemia, which had led me to be hospitalized during my flare-ups in 2008 and 2011, she encouraged me to drink electrolyte water and take an iron supplement. Why had I never thought of that before?

"What are you making?" Ryan asked, looking over my shoulder.

"A chocolate avocado smoothie," I said, pouring some almond milk into the blender. It was a variation on the smoothie I'd had in Southern California during my flare-up after Asher was born. Just like now, I had lost a ton of weight, wasn't able to keep anything down, and had a taste for absolutely nothing—except a chocolate shake. So Ryan and I went to a juice bar where I ordered a chocolate milkshake, but I asked them to prepare it without ice cream or milk. They ended up making me a smoothie with almond milk, peanut butter, chocolate syrup, ice, and a banana. It was amazing. Now that I was trying to make it at home, I substituted raw cacao for the chocolate syrup and almond butter for the peanut butter. I also added half a chilled avocado for some healthy fat. I dropped in some of the L-glutamine Dr. Hestor said would help my gut heal and collagen peptides for extra protein. I had to admit, it felt good to be back in the "lab"—particularly when the result was something that tasted just like a Frosty from Wendy's to me.

I drank one of those shakes at most meals, along with a lot of bone broth and, of course, SCD chicken soup. After giving my body plenty of rest in bed, completely free of any physical strain or the day-to-day stressors of ferrying kids around, cooking, cleaning, running a business, grocery shopping—you name it—I slowly started to recover.

I also started a new protocol of gut-healing anti-inflammatory supplements along with low-dose naltrexone (LDN) to help modulate my immune system. After years of being off the anti-inflammatory medication mesalamine (the glorified Advil for the gut), I restarted that again too. I hated that I had to go back on medication, but my UC was so severe, Ryan and I were starting to realize that sometimes I needed food *plus* a little boost to help turn things around. And that particular drug didn't give me any side effects. Plus I couldn't bear to miss any more time with my boys. And I sensed there was one more thing I should do.

"I feel like I need to tell my followers what's been happening," I confessed to Ryan one night. "I haven't posted any new recipes in months. They're going to start wondering what's wrong." I paused for a moment. I could feel the tears forming. I tried to take a deep breath, but it caught in my throat. As I looked up at Ryan, I felt the first hot tear slide down my cheek. "What am I supposed to say?"

He leaned in, kissed my forehead, and said exactly what I expected: "Just be honest with them. Tell them the truth."

"But—"

"Babe," he quickly cut in, "these people know you. They love you. And one of the things they love about you is that you've always been so open and honest about your health. You've never held back anything before. Don't start now. What you're going through is all part of the journey. Let them see that."

"But what if—"

He held up his hand to stop me, knowing exactly what I was going to say. "They're not going to be upset. Or disillusioned. Or disappointed." He took both my hands in his and looked into my eyes. "They're not going to leave, Danielle."

I so wanted to believe him. And deep down . . . I did. Ryan had always been the voice of reason, articulating realities that my brain knew to be true but my heart and personal insecurity struggled to accept. He was right. This *was* a journey. And it wasn't always going to be pretty. My followers had a right to know that. I suspected a lot of them already did. After all, most of us were on the same journey, battling the same diseases, the same symptoms, the same fears, and the same insecurities. They needed to know that I wasn't any different. That I understood.

I hoped they would understand too.

The next afternoon, I sat down at my laptop and started writing.

This is a hard post to write. Because I vowed in 2011, when Asher was a baby, that this would never happen again. It's also difficult because if I let it, it can make me feel like a failure. If I sit and wallow in my thoughts, I start to blame myself for not being strict enough or not trying hard enough.

You may have noticed that I was pretty quiet on social media and my blog for the month of March and much of April. . . . Unfortunately, I was battling an ulcerative colitis flare-up for a few months and my bandwidth was pretty much taken up by trying to get well and still take care of my family. I looked so unwell that I avoided posting on social media in hopes of not concerning everyone.

I told them about the flare-ups I experienced after each of my pregnancies, and how hard I tried to avoid the same thing happening after Easton's birth. And about the debilitating symptoms that kept me bedridden for almost eight weeks, unable to spend time with or even take care of my own children. I told them about our visit with Dr. York, my refusal to go back on steroids, the elimination diet, the shakes, the soups, and the supplements. Then I got to the part I was dreading the most.

I've spent a lot of time over the past couple of months beating up on myself for not being perfect. . . . I mainly blamed myself, but as I looked closer, I realized there was a lot that led up to this that was out of my control.

I took a deep breath. *Here we go.*

I had been on an anti-inflammatory prescription called mesalamine (Lialda) for many years as a precautionary and maintenance measure since it did not cause any side effects. In the wellness community, Western medicine can be vilified, and we can feel like a failure if we do not achieve health through diet alone. I came to the decision that while it didn't work on its own (I've had many flares while on Lialda without diet), it potentially could be working hand in hand with my diet.

Enter that failure complex—I get hundreds of emails weekly from you all. Testimonies of finding health for various diseases and quitting medications and staying in remission. I have put unnecessary pressure on myself for the past 7 years to try to live med-free just like these wonderful testimonies. After a couple years of feeling well and eating a Paleo diet, I started lowering my dose of Lialda and weaning myself off of it over the course of a year. My body now did not have the anti-inflammatory support from the drug, and I wasn't treating the inflammation naturally. Either way, I needed to support my body with something more than just diet.

I also told them about the antibiotics I had before and after my C-section with Easton and the norovirus that hit our whole family when he was three months old. Then I zeroed in on what I truly believe was at the eye of this latest storm—stress.

If you have an autoimmune disease, you know that stress can be your worst enemy. I've had a ton of stress over the past 2 years. Most of it stems from Aila's death, which transitioned over to my pregnancy with Easton, as well as his well-being and safety after birth. . . . In addition to that, I am a type A person and stress over pretty much everything. I stressed over writing my new book and whether or not everyone would like it, that I wasn't posting enough new recipes on the blog . . . or that Asher wasn't getting enough attention after the new baby arrived.

I described another source of pressure I felt as a new mom, which led to a decision I made that might have pushed my system over the edge.

As moms, we also put so much stress on ourselves to breastfeed. . . . After my [milk] supply decreased from the norovirus, I was so worried about it, I took milk inducing supplements and ate a ton of oats in hopes of it increasing. I believe they caused serious gastrointestinal upset, but my mommy blinders kept me from seeing it because I was only focused on the goal of [producing] more milk. I actually believe these [two things] were the final straw that sent me into the flare, after everything else from above building up.

I love breastfeeding. I think it is one of the most special bonds between a mother and her child. But women are under so much pressure about it. They worry their babies aren't getting enough, or their supply is too low. It's a terrible feeling to feel like you can't provide for your child. I was forced to stop with Asher at 9 months because of my illness, which is still a fantastic amount of time, but I have had guilt about it ever since. I hated that my health forced me to stop, and we didn't make the decision together based on his needs and my needs. I always felt like I was robbed. . . .

Ultimately, I had to realize that "mom" was more important to [Easton] than "mom's milk," and take care of myself first so I could be present for him and Asher.

Don't lose the forest for the trees or in this instance, the baby for the milk. Make sure you are there for your family first, and not pursuing something that may hurt them in the long run.

Being a mom is hard work. Being a working mom can be even harder. Be sure to prioritize your disease, even when you are not in a flare. Take care of yourself, rest, and relax. It's ok to need a break.

I sat back and read what I had written so far. It felt like a lot. I had been candid with my followers before, but never to this extent. It's not that I'd been hiding anything. Social media just never felt like the right place to "get into the weeds" of it all. But now that I saw my entire journey laid out in crisp Filosofia font, somehow it just felt . . . right. At one point, my followers and I were alone—each one of us. We were frightened and struggling to come to terms with diseases and conditions none of us asked for. Yet we found a way to push through. To survive. We found answers. We found hope. We found one another.

I took a moment or two to think and then continued typing.

I started this blog to help others and offer hope. . . . My theory is that I experience these flare-ups to remind me why I am doing what I am doing, and to continue striving to help everyone out there that is going through tragedy, be it health or loss. I believe in healing and do believe I will experience full healing at some point. But for now, I think I'm meant to still "have" this disease and manage the symptoms with diet. So if you're trying, and you're still getting sick here and there—know that there's no such thing as a perfect healing journey, and know you are not alone.

I didn't realize I had started crying until Ryan came in and asked how the post was coming along.

"It's good," I said, sniffling.

"Yeah?" he said, catching my eye.

"Yeah."

"You said everything you want to say?"

I nodded.

"Still a little scared?" he asked, a gentle smile forming.

I nodded. I hated that I was, but I was. I had even included a couple of pictures of me that Ryan had taken over the past few weeks to show how serious my condition had become. And frankly, I looked awful. Skeletal, pale, circles under my eyes, thinning hair—a far cry from the glossy glamour shots my followers were used to seeing in the cookbooks.

I didn't sleep a wink that night, wondering what people were making of the post. How would they react to the revelation that I wasn't making it on food alone? Would they continue to believe that food can make a difference? Would I lose all credibility?

I was still awake when the first rays of morning light started peeking through the blinds. I carefully snuck out of bed so I wouldn't wake Ryan. The house was silent. Both boys were still fast asleep. I crept into the dining room, sat down at the table, and flipped open my laptop.

Okay, Danielle, I said to myself. *Let's see what kind of damage you've done.* I pulled up the post and held my breath as the page loaded. *Did anyone comment?*

They did. Thousands of them, in fact.

Thank you for your raw honesty. You are an inspiration, even for those of us who do not suffer from autoimmune disease.

Danielle, your courage to share helps so many people. We've learned to expect our happily ever after, and when that doesn't

happen, we feel like a failure, when really there is no pure happily-
ever-after without struggle too. Your honesty is a breath of fresh air.

Thank you for making yourself so vulnerable and revealing what
it is like to live with chronic illness . . . the good times and bad
. . . with strangers! . . . It is easy to feel so lonely and isolated
emotionally (even when you clearly know you are not) and so
hard not to go down the road of "I'll never feel better again!" . . .
Thank you for your honesty and for sharing your struggles. . . .
It's a real blessing to others.

This post has actually helped me in feeling less isolated. . . .
Thank you for your vulnerability in sharing such a difficult time
with the world; it is a mark of true strength when you can lift
others up in your own turmoil.

For the second time in less than twenty-four hours, Ryan walked
in to find me crying in front of my computer.

"So . . . ?" he asked tentatively. "How'd they react?"

By this point I was in full-blown ugly-crying mode. So much so
that I couldn't even form words. I just turned my laptop toward Ryan
and let him read the comments for himself.

"See?" he said, wrapping me in a big hug. "I told you they wouldn't
leave."

By the end of the week, more than four thousand people had
commented on the post on my blog or on Facebook—and not one
of them was the least bit negative or critical. I was so worried that
showing my own failures and shortcomings would weaken the community, but if anything, it strengthened it. Emboldened by my confes-
sions, others shared their own fears and insecurities, and the online
community rallied behind them in support. It was the best medicine
I could possibly imagine.

Within a few weeks, I started feeling stronger. Though the flare-up was worse than what I experienced during the first book tour and after Aila's death, it wasn't anywhere near as bad as the one I experienced after Asher was born or the one I had in Africa. Yes, I needed a little help from Western medicine. I also needed rest and a break from all the stress I'd been under. But once again, food had led the way in my recovery. I was beginning to see how all of it was connected. More of the puzzle pieces were starting to line up.

This time I recognized that something else had strengthened me as well: community. No one should ever have to suffer through a disease alone. I was grateful I didn't have to. Now hopefully my followers knew they didn't have to either.

———————

That sense of community drove me as I began work on my fourth cookbook. My publisher and I had agreed that it would focus on comfort foods. Over the years I had received thousands of requests for things that were difficult for the average home cook to convert to healthier versions from their tried-and-true index card recipes, or the tattered hand-me-down cookbooks from their grandmothers.

Among the top requested recipes were meals like chicken pot pie, chicken and dumplings, shrimp and grits, and biscuits and gravy, as well as breads, sides, and snacks like bagels, donuts, onion rings, cheese crackers, and animal crackers. Many people had requested recipes for comforting soups and simple but flavorful dinners, easy stews, and creamy make-ahead casseroles. They also wanted nostalgic treats and desserts like corn dogs, fish sticks, silky cheesecake with blueberry preserves, pineapple upside-down cake, and Girl Scout cookie remakes. And of course, they longed for pizza and fried chicken—every childhood favorite they could remember and now missed. And to be honest, I was with them. Healthy eating aside, those were the foods I missed most too.

"That seems like a lot," Ryan commented one night as he perused my list.

"Yeah," I agreed, "but look on the bright side. The taste tests are going to be out of this world!"

I decided to start with the recipes I first learned how to cook from my mom—the French dip sandwiches and the creamy chicken divan and poppy seed chicken casseroles. I had already created a dairy-free cream of mushroom soup for my Thanksgiving green bean casserole recipe in *Celebrations*, so the rest would be easy.

Once again, my kitchen became a laboratory, where from one delicious tasting after another, I put together an entire cookbook with over a hundred recipes that comforted my soul and that I knew would soothe the soul of anyone who picked up a copy.

The best part was, I was able to share many of my own childhood traditions with my kids—things they had yet to experience because of our special way of eating. For the first time, they were able to munch on hot pizza pockets and warm toaster tarts filled with cinnamon and sugar and coated with a sweet glaze. They finally got to enjoy my mom's creamy casseroles blanketed in silky rich sauces. Not to mention every kid's favorites—cheese crackers, flaky animal cookies, and cold glasses of dairy-free chocolate milk.

Watching the way my kids and generous taste testers devoured and enjoyed the recipes filled me with hope that this might just be my best cookbook yet.

Ironically, about the time I sent the final draft to my publisher in December 2017, I was gearing up to do another round of promotion for my previous cookbook, *Celebrations*. It had released the year before and was filled with recipes for the holidays—providing perfect material for an episode of Hallmark's *Home & Family* just days before Christmas. After I'd spent months experimenting in the kitchen, showcasing a few festive family favorites seemed the perfect way to cap off the year.

14

"So what are you going to make for them?" Ryan asked me over dinner. We were discussing my upcoming appearance on Hallmark's *Home & Family* to plug *Celebrations*. And this year, we had a lot to celebrate ourselves!

Though I had experienced that frustrating flare-up right on cue—nine months after Easton's birth—I'd been able to stay out of the hospital *and* avoid steroids, which was further proof that food was the constant in helping me combat my UC.

Celebrations became my third cookbook to hit the *New York Times* Best Sellers list, and I made my first appearance on the *Today* show. My blog following also continued to expand, which meant that even more people were starting to embrace and reap the benefits of grain-free, gluten-free, dairy-free living.

But without question, our biggest celebration of 2017 came on June 12, when Ryan and I welcomed our daughter, Kezia (Kez-ee-ah)

Elisabeth, to the world. We named her after one of the daughters of the biblical character Job. After suffering a series of devastating losses, including the deaths of all of their children, Job and his wife had ten more children. Job named his second daughter after the sweet-smelling cassia (cinnamon) tree, a reminder that God had brought him through his many trials and made his latter years sweet. A Hebrew verb meaning "It is done" is also connected to the name, so perhaps Job chose this name because he knew his time of suffering had come to an end. It was a name I had written in tiny print on the top right corner of my journal when I was still pregnant with Aila. I wasn't sure I would ever have a chance to use it, or if I would even want to, but it stood out to me and I noted it just in case.

A promise to hope for.

When we found out this baby was a girl, I was terrified to get excited. My ache over losing Aila and the joy I'd had anticipating our mother-daughter bond persisted. But as this pregnancy progressed and my doctor assured me she was healthy, I slowly opened myself to those dreams again.

The moment they placed Kezia in my arms, my heart erupted with love, and a piece of it healed that I wasn't sure would ever heal. I realized that Asher's heart healed that day, too, as he held her for the first time and bent down to kiss her forehead. She was the balm for our hearts we hadn't known we would ever find. And she taught me that it was okay to hope again.

Now six months after Kezia's birth, I still felt good and was heading to *Home & Family* to show the audience that food can be healthy and taste amazing—that we aren't really giving up anything by eating foods that heal us.

"I'm making your favorite," I said, winking at Ryan.

His face lit up. "Short ribs?"

"Yep. The Cabernet-Braised Short Ribs with Parsnip-Turnip Puree." I had included this recipe in the Valentine's Day section of

Celebrations. We both loved these ribs because they're so tender they melt in your mouth.

"Good choice." I knew he'd say that. Ryan *loves* short ribs. Ribs of any sort, really. We used to go to Houston's, a fancy restaurant in the city, on his birthday so he could order a rack of their ribs. But when we began eating differently, short ribs had to go—until I decided to recreate them, coming up with different gluten- and sugar-free sauces, and splurging on 100 percent grass-fed ribs. I had developed several different recipes—one for each of Ryan's birthdays—and whether it was the Thai red curry or the barbecue beef, each was every bit as delicious as the original. I knew that when people thought about "healthy" eating, they probably didn't think of short ribs cooked in luscious red wine. I was excited about shattering that misconception.

Because Hallmark doesn't mess around when it comes to Christmas, I knew the set would be decked out with trees and fake snow, so I took Asher with me to see it. As expected, he was in awe of the dozens of Christmas trees and the artificial snow in the 90-degree heat, just as his Christmas-obsessed mama was. He even got to stand behind the cameras while we filmed the segment, which might have been as much fun for me as it was for him.

That day, I cooked for the two hosts, Debbie Matenopoulos and Mark Steines, along with show regulars Ken Wingard, Paige Hemmis, and Matt Iseman and two guests. Before I started the segment, the group sat behind a countertop overlooking the stove and my work area and began eating their own previously prepared dishes.

"This is fall-off-the-bone delicious," Matt announced, his mouth dripping with sauce.

I smiled politely, but inside I was doing a happy dance.

"I can't do white potatoes because they cause inflammation in my body," I explained as we moved on to the parsnip and turnip puree, "so I do some different root vegetables instead."

"That wasn't mashed potatoes?" Matt blurted out, stunned.

"Nope," I smiled, elated that he hadn't missed the taste of mashed potatoes with milk and butter mixed in.

"Can you believe it?" Debbie remarked.

"I love parsnips," Ken chimed in enthusiastically, "and this is the best parsnip puree I've ever had. They're so light and fluffy."

"Thank you," I said, ready to burst with joy.

After we completed the dish and showed the finished plate, which looked beautiful, Debbie grabbed the bowl of freshly made puree from the food processor and walked it over to Matt. "I'm going to give Matt this right here."

"And how about a little more of that?" he said, pointing to the ribs as he grabbed a spoon and dipped out more of the puree. Then he passed the bowl to Ken, who scraped a nice helping onto his now-empty plate.

The appearance couldn't have gone better. It was awesome watching everyone genuinely enjoy what I had made—in front of a national audience, no less! I knew that every time they commented on how delicious something was, part of them was thinking, *Wait, this has all of this alternative, healthy stuff in it—and it tastes this good?*

And in my mind, I answered back, *Yes, yes, it does!*

———

"I think people are starting to get it," I told Ryan when Asher and I got back home. "You really can eat healthy and not sacrifice any of the taste."

My appearance on *Home & Family* had really put me in the Christmas spirit, and I couldn't wait to spend a relaxing holiday together at home as a family. I savored every last minute of that holiday season, because as good as I had been feeling, I knew what was coming.

I had already resigned myself to the fact that I would have

another flare-up after Kezia's birth. Not only had I had a C-section and course of antibiotics the previous June, I was getting by with little sleep while caring for three young children and working on my fourth cookbook. But a baby whom I would get to love on for life was more than worth any health setback. And my hope had been that I could mitigate some of the symptoms by getting ahead of them.

Then, like clockwork, as soon as I started introducing solid foods to Kezia in early February, my UC symptoms returned. *This is part of the experience; you know that,* I reminded myself. *Just stay focused on getting through it and resting. You have to be well for the release of the next cookbook in December.*

I canceled or postponed any immediate work and travel plans, and started working with Dr. Hestor, my functional medicine MD, who readjusted my supplements to ensure I was receiving enough iron to allow my body to work through the flare and get back to normal as quickly as possible. I put myself on bed rest and took life as slowly and calmly as I could, mentally willing myself not to get stressed out or anxious. I drank those chocolate-banana protein shakes multiple times a day so I wouldn't lose too much potassium or protein.

Still, spending all day in bed can lead to lots of self-deprecation and dark thoughts, and I knew how easily I could fall into the trap of questioning whether food really was the miracle cure I claimed it to be. I needed a reminder. I needed to keep track of my victories. Along with my recipe journals, I had been keeping a food and symptom journal to help me track what I was eating and how I felt afterward during each of my flare-ups. During my last flare with Easton, I'd been so weak I could barely write, so Ryan created an app to make it easier for me. I pulled it up on my phone and reviewed it.

Though multiple bathroom trips were once again part of my experience, I noticed that this time around, I wasn't feeling pain when I went, nor did I have bone or eye pain. My iron levels remained at a near healthy level as well. But for some reason, I just couldn't shake the stubborn flare-up.

I wondered whether that might have been because I had a girl instead of a boy. Perhaps the hormone levels were somehow different. When I raised that possibility with Dr. Veerman, she was unable to confirm it but said it was definitely possible. My counselor also reminded me that a lot of my grief was unearthed during my pregnancy with Kezia, and I hadn't really been processing it or working through it.

I started losing a lot of weight—significantly more than my pregnancy weight gain. I knew enough by this point to keep myself hydrated and make sure I got plenty of protein and potassium in my diet, so I began drinking lots of electrolyte water. But even though I was working hard at getting everything under control, the symptoms wouldn't go away completely.

The hardest part was that I couldn't be the kind of fully present mom I wanted to be. I would gather my strength so we could play games, cuddle in my bedroom, and watch television. When Asher went to school, Easton would bring in his toys so we could play together and watch cartoons. And I had just enough strength to nurse Kezia and hold her close to me.

But in the quiet times, when I lay in bed alone, my inner critic would start in on me, cataloging and criticizing every little slip I made along the way. *I should have been stricter. I shouldn't have had that ice cream at Disneyland. I should have spaced out my travel schedule a little more. Or slept more while Kezia slept. Sleep when the baby sleeps, they say. What's wrong with me? How am I supposed to help other people if I can't even help myself?* And then the tears would come.

"Dani," Ryan reminded me for the umpteenth time, "go easy on yourself. If it wasn't for the way you've been eating, your symptoms would have been much worse, and you probably would have been in the hospital for weeks by now." He lifted my chin so he could look into my eyes. "Right?"

I nodded and wiped at my tears.

"Look at how much your way of eating has helped," he said reassuringly. "Focus on that, okay?"

I tried my best to remain optimistic, and I did see *some* improvement, but when I stepped on the bathroom scale and saw that I had lost nearly ten pounds in just two weeks, I knew it was time to get the medical community involved. I didn't want my weight to plummet twenty or thirty pounds as it had in the past. I knew that was when I usually fell off the proverbial cliff. It would have been negligent to keep waiting for the supplements and food to work on their own. By now I knew my body's limits. I could do only so much. Food and supplements could do only so much. I needed help—before I was too far gone.

"Ryan," I said hesitantly, "I think I need to go see Dr. York."

"Are you sure?" he asked, taking my hand. He knew how desperately I tried to avoid bringing doctors into the mix.

I nodded. "I just don't want a repeat of what I experienced with Asher or with Easton." He agreed, and the next morning, we headed back to my gastroenterologist.

"You know he's going to say prednisone," I said as we walked into the medical building.

"Yeah," Ryan agreed solemnly, "he's going to say prednisone."

And of course, he said prednisone.

Actually, his nurse practitioner said it. Dr. York's schedule was booked, and my symptoms were too severe to wait for an opening. Besides, we already knew what he was going to say. And since he hadn't even examined me during my previous visit, what was the difference?

As I described my symptoms and concerns to the nurse practitioner, I noticed she barely listened, as though she'd already made up her mind. Still . . . it was worth a try.

"You know," I said, "eating the right food has been really helpful in the past, and if at all possible, I'd like to avoid—"

She interrupted me. "You think food really helps?"

Her reaction stunned me for a moment. *That wasn't a criticism. She is actually interested.* I glanced hopefully at Ryan.

"Yeah," I continued. "It actually has *really* made a difference. I've noticed I can control my pain and bleeding with the foods I avoid. But I can't quite seem to get into complete remission."

She nodded, listening intently.

Hey, we're actually getting somewhere! This is great!

She pulled a pen out of her pocket and started scribbling on a pad of paper. I leaned forward to see what she was writing.

"I'm going to start you on forty milligrams of prednisone."

Wait. What? I stared, slack-jawed, at Ryan. He looked equally stunned. But the nurse had been listening. She had acted like she believed me!

She ripped the sheet off the pad and handed it to me. Sure enough, there it was: *prednisone.*

I sighed deeply. "I can't take this drug."

"I'm sorry," she said, "this is all I can do for you."

Desperate, I made a follow-up appointment with Dr. York.

"You know I really don't do well on prednisone," I said to him. "I don't want to take it." I could feel tears stinging my eyes.

"Is there *anything* else we can do?" Ryan pleaded on my behalf.

Dr. York thought for a moment. "Well, there is this other steroid called budesonide. It takes a little longer to work, but there are minimal to zero side effects."

My jaw dropped. Was he serious? No side effects? Why hadn't anybody told me about this steroid in the ten years I'd been dealing with this disease?

"I'd like to try it," I said eagerly.

"Okay," he said, grabbing his pad and pen. "Let's give it a shot."

Ryan and I went straight from the medical building to the pharmacy. Neither of us could remember feeling so hopeful walking out of a doctor's office before. It was further confirmation that I needed to take an active role in my own health and not just blindly accept whatever the doctor ordered. After all, who knew my body, my symptoms, and what my system could and couldn't tolerate better than me?

Dr. York had been right. The budesonide took a little longer to kick in, but within ten days, I was able to get out of bed. This new medication was like a booster, activating the healing process that the food and supplements had already laid the groundwork for. It wasn't long before my symptoms subsided completely—and without any side effects.

Within a month, I decided it was time to start weaning myself off the drug. When I first started taking it, I had stopped nursing Kezia for fear that the budesonide might get into her system through my milk. I even "pumped and dumped" multiple times a day to keep my supply up. But now that the flare was over, I was anxious to get back to nursing.

I half-expected Dr. York to lecture me on what a terrible decision I'd made, but then he surprised me again.

"You don't need to wean off those," he said. "You can just cut them."

No side effects. No weaning period. Honestly, where had this steroid been all my life?

Despite his advice, I stopped them gradually. If nothing else, I figured it would be good for my body to ease into controlling the inflammation naturally after depending on the meds to do it for several weeks. I still hated that I had to use medication, but at least this time, the solution didn't feel worse than the problem. And if it helped me get back to my kids more quickly, then I was grateful for it.

———————

Once again, life felt good. My symptoms now gone, I was able to focus on being the best mom I could be and on teaching my children to love food as much as I enjoyed and embraced it.

I think a lot of people with food sensitivities worry about their kids not adapting to a new palate of tastes and textures, but I've actually found the opposite to be true. Easton had pretty much always eaten healthy (though he's the kind of kid who would probably shove half the bag of candy in his mouth while you are looking the other way), but Asher had to learn. I had started out feeding him what most moms do—the cereals, the puffs, fish-shaped cheese crackers, the works. But one year while listening to a panel of women who ate like I did talk about how their kids ate what they did, I realized something: If it was important to my own body to get healthy nourishment, wouldn't it be even more important for a young, growing little body? A doctor on the panel also mentioned that children of parents with autoimmune diseases were more likely to inherit it, and worse, babies born via C-section were more likely to have allergies and autoimmune diagnoses. All of my kids were cesarean babies.

I returned from that conference with new resolve. No more processed foods with gluten and sugar in them. Now Asher doesn't see the way our family eats as weird, bad, or "less than." It's just the way we eat. And he loves it. I'm grateful that I wasn't trying to switch a teenager from regular pasta to spaghetti squash, but it's still a chore, no matter the age.

At the start of the school year, I'd asked Asher's teacher to let me know when special events were coming up so I could offer him an alternative that would allow him to have fun and enjoy the event without feeling left out. So when he came home one afternoon with a note telling me that his class was having a party with cupcakes at the end of the week, I got down at his eye level and said, "What kind of cupcake do you want to take with you for your party this week?"

Asher's eyes lit up. "Chocolate!" Then he grew serious. "But Mom, can I eat some of the icing off the other kids' cupcakes?"

I laughed and tussled his hair. "Yes, you can do that."

If eating the icing off a friend's cupcake would make Asher feel more normal, I was okay with it. My goal was to make sure he understood *why* we eat differently, so that one day, when he is grown up, he will make his own healthy choices. Plus, I knew he'd likely take two bites of frosting and discard the rest of the cupcake. He just wasn't used to that much sugar.

"He probably won't even like it," I told Ryan that night.

Like all kids, mine prefer some things over others and refuse to eat some things, period. But as far as they're concerned, our meals and snacks are just food—delicious, sweet, crunchy, chewy, savory, flavorful food.

———————————

Eat What You Love: Everyday Comfort Food You Crave was set to go on sale six months after Kezia's first birthday. I couldn't wait for the release. We had planned a completely different, cutting-edge tour that I knew the Against All Grain following would love, complete with live cooking demos, meet and greets where I would get to hear their stories and hug everyone who had supported me over the years, cocktail hours, special guest interviews, and Q&A sessions.

"I'm just going to say it again," Ryan said, looking at the proposed itinerary. "This seems like a lot."

I knew he was worried. So was I. As invigorating as this tour promised to be, it was also going to be exhausting. My plan? To mitigate the stress with down days between stops, get as much sleep as possible, and eat really well along the way. We also cut the number of stops in half from previous tours.

As part of the media tour, I got to make a repeat appearance on the *Today* show. Actually, I felt as if my connection with this program went way back. The producer I'd found after searching online for hours and then sending information to random email addresses had declined my guerilla marketing pitch when *Against All Grain* released in 2013. But I wasn't one to take no for an answer. When I was in New York for my first book signing tour, I woke up at 5:00 a.m. (which was actually 2:00 a.m. Pacific time!) to go down to the plaza and hand-deliver copies to the hosts when they came out to greet fans. Let me tell you, lugging six five-pound cookbooks through the streets of New York City was no easy feat!

I arrived just as the hosts were coming outside. As soon as they got within shouting distance, I shamelessly called them over and handed them each their own copy, hoping they wouldn't toss them aside once they got back in the studio. Because so many people were there, I didn't get a chance to make a pitch, so my recipes would have to speak for themselves.

I had struck up a conversation with a woman and her daughter who were standing next to me along the barricade. She later reached out to me on Facebook to tell me that Al Roker had sent a producer back out to find me, but I had already left. I don't know what would have come of that if I'd stayed, but I always felt as if I missed my chance. I was invited on when *Celebrations* released, but my segment was rushed and I was a little nervous.

Now, finally, five years and three cookbooks after my near-encounter with Al Roker, I was getting my real chance. My segment was longer than normal, and all three hosts were there, plus I was able to showcase two different recipes.

I had decided to make shrimp fried rice and snickerdoodle cookies to demonstrate both a savory and a sweet option.

Just like Matt Iseman at the Hallmark taping, Hoda Kotb dug into the dish before the segment even started. I knew Hoda ate dairy-free, so she was really the one I was hoping to impress.

"This is so good," mumbled Howie Mandell, who was sitting in as a guest host that day, his mouth full of "rice."

"Good!" I smiled. "Do you miss the rice?" I asked, referring to the cauliflower rice I used in place of regular rice.

"No," he said, shaking his head. "I don't miss anything!"

"Don't leave the shrimp!" chirped Kathy Lee Gifford as she ran back to eat the leftovers out of the pan.

The segment was going even better than I had expected, and we hadn't even gotten to the egg-free, gluten-free, dairy-free snickerdoodles yet. That, I knew, would be the real test. After all, snickerdoodles were a holiday classic. Everyone knew exactly what they were supposed to taste like. Buttery-soft on the inside, snickerdoodles are famous for their cracked and crispy outside and intense flavor from the cinnamon and sugar they're rolled in before baking. But in my version, I also put cinnamon *into* the dough to give it an extra-spicy punch. I used maple sugar instead of the traditional refined white sugar to give the cookies a nice crunch with a subtle maple flavor. Unfortunately, we ran out of time before I could talk about them, but Hoda grabbed a quick bite and said they were delicious. The way the rest of the cast and crew gobbled down the rest told me I had nailed the recipe.

———

By early 2019, I was in full swing—working, mothering, traveling, blogging, and beginning to create recipes for my next cookbook. I knew it was a lot to take on, but I was confident that my body could handle it. I shared my final, sweet nursing session with Kezia a week before leaving for tour, knowing that I wouldn't want to keep pumping on the road for a mere four to six ounces a day.

As I began the book tour for *Eat What You Love*, the highlight, as always, was getting to meet and hear the stories of people who were using my recipes to find relief from their own symptoms.

One woman approached me at a signing and told me, through tears, that she had tried to get pregnant for ten years and couldn't—even with fertility treatments—because of a thyroid issue. I listened intently as she shared her frustrations, remembering how terrified I had once been that my disease might keep me from having the family I so desperately wanted. Then she introduced me to her six-month-old daughter, and we held up the line for five minutes, hugging and crying together.

I met another mom whose eight-year-old son was nonverbal and exhibited behaviors associated with the autism spectrum. She told me she bought one of my cookbooks on the recommendation of a friend who saw a difference in the behavior of her own son after he began eating my recipes.

"How's your son doing?" I asked.

"He's thriving!" she beamed. "He's in a mainstream elementary school with only a part-time special aid."

The most miraculous encounter was with a woman who came to one of my meet-and-greet events. When she approached me, she had a slight limp. I didn't think much of it until I noticed that she was surrounded by family members, all of whom were near tears. As soon as she opened her mouth to speak, she broke down crying. I gave her a gentle hug and told her, "It's okay. I know." I assumed she was struggling with arthritis. I had experienced some pretty severe bone and joint pain myself after giving birth to Asher, so I recognized the gait.

When she finally collected herself enough to speak, she informed me that until recently, she had been using a wheelchair due to severe multiple sclerosis. Then she started using my recipes and following fellow author Dr. Terry Wahls's protocol for MS.

"We didn't think she'd ever be able to stand again, let alone walk," one of her family members explained. "But look . . ." The woman's voice cracked as she gestured at her sister, standing and walking under her own power—no wheelchair, no walker, no cane, no assistance.

"It's all because of food," her other sister said, smiling through tears. "Your food."

It was all I could do to get through the rest of the meet and greet without collapsing under the weight of it all. I had received hundreds of thousands of emails and letters over the years from people who were using food to lessen the symptoms of chronic diseases, but for someone to go from being wheelchair bound to walking under her own power through diet alone? *And to think that I had anything at all to do with it. . . .* It was just too much.

At the end of each night, I held a Q&A and testimonial time, and I asked this woman for permission to repeat her story from the stage. I hoped that from her experience, others would gain the confidence to give their own testimony to the group and hopefully inspire someone else. After she agreed, I shared what she'd told me, and the relief and hope I saw wash over the audience's faces was palpable.

That night when I got back to my hotel room, I plopped down on my bed and started reading some of the cards and letters people had handed me throughout the day. As tired as I was, their stories reenergized me. I read until I fell asleep atop my tear-stained pillow.

The next morning, it all started up again—early flights, back-to-back events, a two-hour stage show of cooking and interviewing followed by signings and meet and greets until 10 p.m. For about two weeks of the tour, I fought through a terrible head cold, so I self-prescribed cold medications and supplements to try to beat it. (For instance, I took lots of elderberry, which is often recommended for colds and flu but can sometimes be difficult for those with autoimmune diseases—something I didn't realize then.) I took special care to get as much sleep as possible, and I ate an incredibly simple and strict diet every night (not even a taste of the amazing samples of my recipes that the caterers prepared each night!), but the adrenaline high of the night and the stories from the audience always kept me up past midnight. It was amazing but exhausting.

Then after the very last event of my tour, I got back to my hotel room late at night and went to the restroom. Blood.

And it wasn't my time of the month. My stomach tensed up. I just needed to get home.

When my flight took off the next morning, I was anxious but fortunately managed to fall asleep about two hours in. When we landed, I felt more relaxed and breathed a deep sigh of relief. But I had also woken up to a harsh reality—I was heading into another flare-up. And so soon after the last.

15

"Do you think you should cut back on your schedule?" Ryan suggested when I got home. "Maybe you didn't fully recover from the minor flare last year, and then all of this book release travel fueled things again."

He had a point. And yet . . .

"How can I? Here," I said, handing him one of the letters I'd received while on the road. "Look at this."

> *Danielle, I'm sure you have days when you're on the road and missing your family and wondering why on earth you're doing this . . . Well, please know that you are making a huge difference in so many lives! Please don't stop!*

"Dan," he said dejectedly. "You can't—"

"And look," I said handing him another one. This is from a seven-year-old, Ryan—*seven!*"

My name is Angela and I am 7 years old. I have Crohn's. My mommy uses all your cookbooks, and I love your recipes. My new favorite is your strawberry popsicles. I want to be just like you and write my own cookbook when I'm older. Then I want to open my own grain-free bakery. I practice by copying your recipes and helping my mom cook. My mom said if you come to our city we could go see you. I hope you come soon!

"How can I say no to that?" The look on his face told me he wasn't budging. "Listen," I assured him. "I'll be fine. I know I've taken on a lot, but if it starts to get bad, I'll just go back on the elimination diet and get it back under control. I've done it before. I can do it again." *There*, I thought, *I almost convinced myself.*

But Ryan wasn't having it. "Danielle, this is what you tell yourself every time, and then it gets you—every time."

"I know," I countered. "But this is different. I have more control over it now."

Ryan just shook his head. We agreed to take a wait-and-see approach. I stuck like glue to my curated mix of the SCD, GAPS, and autoimmune Paleo protocol diets that had worked for me in the past. I also did my best to take it easy and get plenty of rest. By the time summer rolled around, however, I still wasn't feeling 100 percent. It seemed like I was keeping a full-on flare at bay, but if I slipped the tiniest bit, I would go off that cliff again. So I begrudgingly made an appointment with Dr. York.

"When was the last time you had a colonoscopy?" he said, looking down at my file.

"In 2008," I said. "But do we really need to do that? I'm already on the strict elimination diet. And when I had that colonoscopy, I ended up in a flare much worse than when I came in."

"I know it's not pleasant, Danielle," he said sympathetically, "but a colonoscopy is the only thing that will help us see what's really going on in there. Don't forget, your risk of colon cancer is higher because of the UC as it is, plus your risk increases after you've had the disease for more than ten years. And it's been eleven years since you were last scoped."

He certainly painted a grim picture. Still I believed in the elimination diet. It had worked before. It would work again. It just needed more time. My next road tour wasn't until September, which meant I still had a few more months to get everything back under control. And I didn't want to get the procedure and detonate the bomb. "I'll think about it," I conceded.

I stuck to a strict SCD and Paleo diet throughout the summer and early fall, and by the time the tour was ready to kick off, I felt confident I could handle it. Besides, this tour was different. I was going to be spending two weeks on the road, on a bus (no early flights!) with two of my best friends, Angie and Annie, and we were going to be speaking to churches full of women every night.

I knew there was a place for my message of healing through food in the church community because I used to be one of those women in the audience—the one who was raised to believe that whatever we asked for in prayer, we would receive.

When I was little, my family and I would pull into a parking lot, and on cue my mom would say, "Kids, pray for a parking spot!" And we *did* always find a parking spot—eventually. We also prayed for our colds to get better. And they did . . . just like most colds do. Because our prayer requests always seemed to work, I grew up figuring all my prayers would automatically be answered—until they weren't. Or so I thought.

When I first became sick, I asked God for healing—repeatedly. And when my symptoms didn't automatically disappear, I figured I must have done something wrong, or worse, that God wasn't listening. When I was pregnant with Aila, I begged and pleaded for her healing. And it didn't happen.

It took years of feeling deserted and abandoned, questioning, losing and regaining my faith to realize that God was listening. I was sure he had answered some of my prayers. Just not the way I expected.

God didn't miraculously heal me. Instead, he placed people in my path—Dr. Stark, Dr. Walters, Jeanine, Susan's daughter, Becky—to help me learn how to help heal myself. And look what that led to! I wanted the women attending these events to hear that sometimes God wants us to come alongside him and take an active role in our own healing so that we can be better prepared to help others. I also wanted them to hear that over the years I had struggled with a lot of doubt and feelings of abandonment. And that it is okay to be working through those for however long you need to. I mean, I'm still working through them. I haven't found all the answers. I assume some questions—like why Aila died—will never be answered on earth. But I have learned to persevere so I can see the light within my dark tunnel, not just at the end of it. That was a message I believed in, and one that I was eager to share.

I had been to too many conferences where the women speakers seemed as if they had it all together. Like they never doubted or questioned. And it always left me feeling less than. I wanted to show these women my real struggles.

So I took every precaution to make sure I would be okay. I whipped up a massive batch of SCD chicken soup before we left and brought it on the bus with us. That's all I ate, three times a day, every day—even when the sweet church staff prepared gluten-free food for me and the crew. I committed to retiring to my bunk immediately after the programs to get some rest, even if everyone else was having a blast chatting until midnight. And I was armed with my arsenal of supplements, which I stored in that bunk.

After the first full week on the road, I was supposed to fly home to be with my kids for two days before returning for our second leg. Unfortunately, my body had already started to decline a bit, and I knew that the back-to-back four-and-a-half-hour flights would likely do me in—not to mention the emotional stress of seeing my kids for only one day and then having to say goodbye again. So I made the difficult decision to stay in Nashville and rest. Fortunately Ryan was working from home at the time, and his parents came over to help nearly every evening. While it might have been the best thing for my health, it was brutal. Thirteen days was the longest I had ever been away from my kids. We talked over FaceTime every evening on the bus. Asher would tell me about things he and his friends did at school, Easton would bring me up to speed on all his favorite cartoons, and Kezia would just chatter happily away about nothing and everything from the comfort of Ryan's arms. It was wonderful seeing their little faces, but I hated being away from them for even one night.

I will never travel this long again, I vowed.

———

I finally got home on October 1 after sharing my message of hope and healing with thousands of women all over the South. My health had declined a lot during the two weeks on tour, but now that I was home, I focused all my energy on getting better. *Food and rest—that's what I need.*

To Ryan's delight, I canceled all my work engagements and spent most of my time in bed. The one thing I couldn't resist was my children. If they were involved in a school function or other fun activity, I forced myself to get up and enjoy it with them. I had already missed a few weeks of their lives; I had no intention of missing out on one minute more. After the event was over, however, I immediately returned to bed, exhausted.

But even though I was sleeping hours upon hours, lying low, and eating only chicken soup, I kept going downhill.

Then one night the kids came into my bedroom to kiss me goodnight. When it was Asher's turn, he looked at me very seriously.

"How long will you be in bed?" he asked. "Will it be like after Kezia was born?"

"I'm not sure, sweetie," I said, touching his cheek. "But we're going to beat this one, and it won't be long."

He looked at me solemnly. "Are you going to die?"

I could hear my own heart shattering. It broke me that my nine-year-old carried such a heavy burden of fear. He knew death intimately since his sister Aila hadn't come home from the hospital. But until now, I didn't realize he remembered me being sick.

"No, sweetie. Mom isn't going to die," I said, trying to keep the quiver out of my voice. "I'm going to get better; it's just taking a little more time." So much for my resolve when he was ten months old that I would never have to utter those words to him.

He stared at me a few seconds longer, and I hoped against all hope he couldn't see my eyes welling up with tears. In so many ways, he was his daddy's little boy—trying to put on a brave front. Yet he was also worrying himself sick—over me. He may have absorbed Ryan's strength, but he'd also inherited my empathy.

I. Hate. This. Disease.

"Come on, buddy," Ryan mercifully broke in. "Let's go to bed and let Mommy get some rest." Hands on Asher's shoulders, he shuffled our son toward the door. "You can play together in the morning."

I figured we'd navigated that okay, but then Asher broke free from Ryan. He ran back to the bed, wrapped his arms around my neck, and kissed me on the cheek. "Please get better, Mom. I love you."

That was it. I was done. The next day, I went back on the budesonide that I had stashed in the back of the medicine cabinet. I *hated* resorting to steroids, but after Asher's plea, I didn't feel as though I had a choice. I could not do this to my family again. I would not. My son could not fear for his mother's life.

This time, however, the budesonide wasn't working. Neither were the chocolate shakes with collagen or the bone broth. *Nothing* that had worked before did this time. I continued to see my functional doctor, Dr. Hestor, who adjusted and readjusted my supplements in an attempt to level out my iron and potassium levels, but with no tangible success. I was growing more and more nauseated, and it was difficult to keep any food down. Unable to stomach anything, I drank electrolyte water as though I'd been stranded in the desert for months. My horrific abdominal pain and the internal bleeding in my colon, which I'd once controlled through food—or the lack thereof—were still frequent and prevalent.

By the end of October, I knew I was getting close to the edge of my cliff. I was losing weight, and I couldn't leave the house for anything except experimental hyperbaric chamber appointments, which I'd started at my functional doctor's recommendation to try to promote healing in my colon and reduce inflammation. I had dark circles under my eyes, and I barely had enough energy to pull myself out of bed.

"I know you don't want to hear this," Dr. York said over the phone, his voice grim, "but given that the budesonide isn't working, I'm afraid you'll need to go back on the prednisone."

I looked at Ryan and nodded forlornly, the phone still pressed to my ear. Even though we'd both known this would be his answer before we called, hearing the words uttered out loud still made my heart sink.

When Ryan got back from the pharmacy, I held that little prescription bottle in my hands and sobbed. *How did everything go so wrong so fast?* I just couldn't understand why none of my tried-and-true remedies were working this time.

"Have I forgotten something?" I asked Ryan.

"Actually, I think you have," he said, grabbing my laptop off the nightstand. He sat down on the edge of the bed and started scrolling. "Remember this?" he said, turning the screen so I could see it.

I expected to see an old symptom journal entry highlighting a specific supplement I'd forgotten to take this time, or a step in the elimination diet I'd somehow omitted. Instead, he had pulled up an Instagram post from the previous year—the one I'd written during my postpartum flare with Kezia.

"But I didn't have to go on prednisone after Easton or Kezia. It's been a decade since I've had to take it." I sighed, still holding the unopened bottle.

"Just read what you wrote," he said, gesturing toward the screen. Next to a photo of me holding Kezia, I'd written:

> Today marks 3 weeks straight in bed with no more than 10 minutes at a time out of my room. Visits from my babies were highlights of my days, and I've watched far too much on Netflix.
>   I'll admit I was frustrated and discouraged to have to resort to strong medication, after so many years of managing with diet, supplements, and lifestyle. But sometimes they're necessary to be able to get to a point where you can reset, and being mom to my kids and a partner to Ryan rather than isolated in bed any longer was more important.

I *had* forgotten that. It was advice I had given my readers after admitting that I had started taking the steroid budesonide to help regulate my symptoms. I understood the fear of side effects as well as the crippling guilt and intense feeling of failure that came with having to turn to modern medicine for help after experiencing success without it. But I didn't want my readers to suffer the consequences of waiting too long to seek pharmaceutical help when necessary as I had. And as I found myself doing now.

I looked up at Ryan, fully prepared to explain why my own advice somehow didn't apply to me, but he cut me off before I could even get the words out.

"Keep reading," he said, scrolling down a little further.

> There are always occasional bumps on the road when you're battling an autoimmune disease, but you just have to keep your eyes on the horizon and keep pushing forward to the smooth and straight parts.

I looked down at the little white, bitter Tic Tac–size pill in my hand and sighed. Ryan was right. (Well … actually, *I* was right.) I just didn't want to admit it. Clearly my system needed more than food to turn itself around. The momentum of this flare was just too great.

"I'm sorry," I said quietly.

"Sorry for what?" Ryan asked, his face a mask of concern.

"You told me I was doing too much, that I needed to slow down— take a break—and I didn't listen. I just thought—"

"I know," he said hugging me gently. "I know."

It was more than an hour before I could actually bring myself to put that pill into my mouth. My own advice aside, I still hated that it had come to this, and I dreaded the side effects I knew would follow, but I just couldn't shake that image of Asher standing by my bed asking if I was going to die. *If this is what it takes for me to be there for my kids*, I resolved as I washed the pill down with some electrolyte water, *this is what I'll do.*

Two days later, I awoke to near darkness.

"Ryan?" I shot up in bed. "Ryan?"

"What's wrong?" came a frantic voice from the doorway.

"I can't see," I said, nearly hysterical. "I can't see anything."

"Don't panic," Ryan cautioned me. "You had trouble with your eyes once before, remember?"

"Not like this!" I could practically feel my heart in my throat. The next thing I heard was Ryan on the phone asking to speak to Dr. York right away. "It's an emergency." Seconds later, he was describing my symptoms to the doctor. All I could hear was the occasional "Uh-huh" and "Okay," followed by "You're sure?" and "Okay, thank you."

"Good news," Ryan said optimistically. "Dr. York said this is somewhat common. He's going to lower your prednisone dosage to 30 milligrams, and that should take care of it."

It turns out Dr. York was right. Lowering the dosage *did* correct the temporary blindness. Unfortunately, it made my other symptoms even worse. So I went back to the 40 milligrams and stayed in bed with my eyes closed, listening to podcasts on my iPhone, waiting for the temporary vision blips to pass. *Honestly*, I thought. *What next?*

"Aren't you coming with us?" my little ballerina princess asked me, her big, brown, doe eyes peeking up over the top of the bed.

"I really wish I could, Kez," I said, brushing a strand of hair out of her eyes. It was Halloween, and Ryan was taking the kids out trick-or-treating—while I lay in bed at home. I could hear Asher and Easton in the background. Both of them were dressed as stick figures, wearing black bodysuits with glow-in-the-dark tape strips for the lines.

"Mommy isn't feeling well enough," I explained gently. "Daddy's going to take you, though, and you can tell me all about it afterward, okay?"

The look on her face broke my heart. When Asher was a baby, I had worried most about missing out on special events—holidays, sports, and school plays. Now here I was. And in August, we had moved just a few miles away to a new home to be in a neighborhood that was filled with young families. I had been so looking forward to the first time trick-or-treating here as a family.

A few days later, I started vomiting uncontrollably. Because I was unable to keep anything down, Ryan took me to the emergency room so I could get some intravenous fluids.

I cried the entire ride over.

"We just need to get some fluids in you, Danielle," Ryan said, trying his best to reassure me. "That's all."

Please, God, I prayed, leaning my head against the cool passenger seat window, *let him be right.*

Shortly after we arrived, Ryan called Dr. York, who came straight down to the ER. Within seconds, he dashed every hope I'd had of going back home that evening.

"I know you've been fighting really hard to get healthy, Danielle, and I commend you for what you've accomplished—I really do," he began.

Don't say it.

"But you're severely anemic and completely dehydrated."

Don't say it.

"I'm going to need to admit you to the hospital. We need to get you on an IV and perform a colonoscopy immediately."

"A colonoscopy?" Ryan said. "Why?"

"Given the severity of her symptoms, I have to be sure she doesn't have colon cancer."

Cancer? I closed my eyes to hold back the tears that threatened to come at any second. I felt like I was trapped in a nightmare I couldn't wake up from.

"Danielle," Dr. York said, his eyes and voice filled with genuine compassion, "I know this isn't what you want, but I'm afraid we're out of options. In addition to the dehydration and anemia, your oxygen levels and blood pressure are abnormally low, and your heart rate is abnormally high. If we don't act now"—he paused for a second—"you may lose your colon."

I squeezed Ryan's hand. As much as it pained me to admit it, deep down I knew he was right. I hadn't been this sick since we were in

Uganda, when I was literally within days of dying. Losing my colon would be horrific. But losing my life? Not being able to be there for my kids? To see them grow up? That was unimaginable. One look at the anguish on Ryan's face told me he was thinking the same thing.

"Okay," I said.

An hour later, I was officially admitted to the hospital—the same one I'd had to go to when Asher was a baby. I felt utterly defeated. I hadn't been hospitalized for this disease in a decade. *I suppose that's something to be proud of*, I thought. I could feel the tears forming again.

This was just a minor setback, I told myself. I'd let modern medicine step in to get my overtaxed system back to where food could take over again. Then I could get back to my kids, back to my work, and back to my sweet husband, who was shouldering so much.

"Okay, Mrs. Walker," the orderly chirped, as he wheeled me into my room. "Let's get you settled in."

Don't worry, Danielle, I thought, forcing a smile, *you'll just be here for a couple of days. You'll be back home again before you know it.*

16

"I just don't understand it," I said to Ryan as he helped me settle into my hospital room. "I mean, I've had flare-ups before—this has never been a smooth road—but I've been able to manage them with food and supplements. Until now."

"I know," Ryan said as he adjusted my pillows.

"I'm proud of what I've learned and accomplished."

"You should be, Dan. You've done an amazing job handling this on your own."

"So what's the problem this time?" I asked, falling back into the bed. "I can't blame it on being postpartum. Kez hasn't nursed in nearly a year. What could I have done wrong? I've been good; I've followed all the protocols that have worked in the past."

"I don't know, babe." He looked every bit as lost as I felt.

After Ryan left to pick up some personal items for me at home and check in on the kids at my parents' house, I tried to figure out—again—what could have led to such a serious flare. I had stopped nursing Kezia in December 2018, right before my January book tour and the start of this flare. Could the cause have been two-fold? I wondered whether another hormonal shift, paired with heavy travel and stress, could have led to an imbalance that just never fully resolved itself. Had I run myself into the ground and not given my body the time it needed to recover from the first tour before heading out on another one in the fall? Could all the immune-boosting supplements I had taken during my bout with influenza A early in the year have activated my immune system? Maybe thrown it into overdrive? Had I accidently ordered something with gluten in it? I just didn't know.

While I was desperately trying to make sense of it all, the nurse came in with her cart full of IV bags and drip lines. She hung them on the metal poles at the head of my bed and then drew the lines to my arm. I turned my head and held my breath when she inserted the needle. I couldn't stand that this was happening to me again.

"Don't you worry, Mrs. Walker. We'll get some fluids and potassium in you, and you'll feel like a new person before you know it," she said.

Before she left my room, she turned and said, "By the way, make sure you have your husband bring your own food in for you. The hospital meals could make things worse. He can bring you bone broth from home. We can keep it in the fridge up here and have one of the nurses reheat it for you."

I looked at her, confused and a bit embarrassed. It was fairly normal for people to recognize me when I was out and about—especially in our hometown—but I looked absolutely horrendous *and* was in a hospital gown. Honestly, I was hoping to fly under the radar. I didn't want anyone to see me like this—so frail and defeated.

"I have all of your cookbooks," she told me, as if reading my expression. "You've really helped me improve my health. Don't worry. You're going to get through this. You'll be home in no time." She smiled and winked.

"Thanks." I smiled back. "I hope so."

Later that evening my phone rang. Ryan was calling on FaceTime. *My babies!*

"Hi, Mom," Asher said, his precious little face marred by a worried expression.

"Hi, Bugs, I miss you!"

"Let me talk to her!" Easton said off camera.

"In a minute," Asher said, brushing his brother away.

"How was school today?"

"Okay. When are you coming home?"

"Soon. Probably in just a couple of days. I'll be home before you know it. I promise."

After visiting briefly with all of them and telling them I loved them, I hung up the phone. I leaned back against the thin hospital pillow and let the tears flow freely.

"I want to be home," I whispered. *I miss my babies and the comfort of my own bed.* I wanted to snuggle with my kids and tuck them in. But instead I lay alone in the semidarkness of my room and listened to the sound of the IV clicking.

The next day Ryan came to visit. "How are you feeling?"

"A little better," I admitted. "Of course, it took three full bags of potassium and a night on saline." I was so sick of talking about sickness. "How are the kids?"

"Okay," he smiled weakly. "But they miss you."

That was the hardest part. Because the kids had been fighting winter colds, the doctors advised that they not come in to see me. My immune system was already compromised; if I were to catch anything from them, it could be catastrophic.

Not only that, but I didn't want them to see their mama hooked up to a ton of wires and tubes in such a foreign and sterile room.

True, I have always believed that it's good to let our kids see us when we're weak, grieving, upset, or even sick. I want them to learn that it's not only okay but it's also healthy to feel emotions. And to learn resilience. But this was too far for me. I didn't want Asher to feel even more concern over whether I would live or die.

"Hang in there," Ryan said, rubbing my free hand. "Just a couple of days and you'll be out of here."

"I know," I said, weaving my fingers through his. I just had to get through the colonoscopy in two days and I'd be home free.

The colonoscopy was a nightmare. As soon as the test was over, my system plummeted. I couldn't tolerate any food or liquids. The bleeding seemed to increase twofold, and I had to make four times as many trips to the bathroom. I also experienced excruciating pain from all the air and the camera that had been inserted, not to mention the gas that filled my colon after its microbiome had been obliterated by the colonoscopy prep and the preliminary round of antibiotics.

On the upside, they *were* able to determine that I did not have colon cancer, a huge relief.

"Well, at least that's a silver lining," Ryan said. "And as soon as your system recovers from the colonoscopy, you'll be able to come home." I loved Ryan's eternal optimism. What I didn't love was the fact that I had to recuperate from a procedure that was supposed to help me. I'd never had to "recover" from a cooking mishap. Sure, before I got the measurements right, I'd get the occasional oily banana loaf or runny snickerdoodle, but I never had to "recover" from eating them. Even my mac and cheese—as horrendous as it was—didn't cause me physical pain. *Chalk up yet another win for food.*

Forty-eight hours later, not only had I not recovered, I felt a hundred times worse than I had when I was admitted.

"I think we should consider putting you on Entyvio," Dr. York said. "I'm very concerned about how bad this flare-up is and what it's doing to your colon."

"But you've definitely ruled out cancer, right?" Ryan asked.

"Yes," Dr. York conceded, "but—" there always seemed to be a *but* when it came to my condition—"the scope showed incredible amounts of inflammation throughout the entire colon."

He turned to me. "I know how you feel about medications— especially ones as strong as this—but here's the reality, Danielle. If you don't go on it, you will likely lose your colon. Entyvio is a biologic that should help control the inflammation in your colon by limiting the number of white blood cells that enter your GI tract. It would address your other symptoms too. We've seen really great results with patients like you."

After Dr. York had finished his explanation, Ryan and I promised to discuss it and get back to him the following day when he came in for his next rounds.

"Considering all the side effects you're having on prednisone, maybe this is the best option right now," Ryan pointed out. "And Dr. York did say that Entyvio wouldn't shut down your body's entire immune system like the steroids or some of the other biologic drugs would. It would target only the white blood cells associated with the inflammation in your colon."

"It would be great not to have to worry as much about catching everything the kids bring home from school," I agreed. Suddenly I remembered something and frowned.

"What is it?" Ryan asked.

"Becky was on a biologic, and I don't think she reacted well to it," I said. I wasn't sure how she was doing now. She and her family had moved out of state a few years before, and I hadn't talked to her since then.

"Well, there are a number of biologics. Remicade, for one," Ryan said. After glancing up at the wall clock, he said, "Listen, I need to go pick up Asher and get the kids dinner. Why don't we do a little more research and talk again later tonight?"

After he left, I grabbed my phone. *What did Becky tell me about biologics?*

I messaged her on Instagram. Not long afterward, she replied. It turns out she had responded poorly to the first biologic she tried, but she had switched to Entyvio about four years earlier. That had made all the difference. Becky said she hadn't had a flare-up since, and she could now eat anything she wanted.

Encouraged, I headed to another website and clicked through to a few patient testimonies. Later that night, I called Ryan to tell him what I'd discovered. "Becky and a lot of other people on Entyvio say they've been in remission for years. Plus, they can eat anything they want."

"Would you actually do that?" Ryan asked.

It was a good question. I had to admit that the thought of eating out without worrying about accidentally getting "glutened" was appealing, not to mention the prospects of being able to splurge occasionally while on vacation or around holidays. But even though I had originally developed recipes to control my symptoms, I really did love the food! I loved eating healthy. And now that I understood more about inflammation and the impact that certain foods have on the digestive system—both good and bad—it was almost impossible to consider *not* eating this way.

"Becky told me she still follows the Paleo/SCD protocol about 80 percent of the time because she knows how good it is for her body," I told him. All symptoms and diagnoses aside, it was just a better, healthier way to eat—and live. "No, I could never go back to eating the way I used to. Not knowing everything I know now."

The next morning, we told Dr. York that we wanted to move forward with the Entyvio. We were encouraged not only by the possibility of fear-free eating, but also by the majority of the testimonials we read, which said that the treatment helped people keep their symptoms under control without the negative side effects of steroids. All things considered, it seemed to be our best option. And my only priority in that moment was returning to my kids as the healthy, vibrant mom they remembered. Whatever was necessary to get me there, right away, was what I wanted.

Unfortunately, our insurance company didn't agree. They wanted us to wait until I was released before I started treatments.

"But don't I *need* the treatments in order to be released?" I asked an equally frustrated Dr. York.

"I'll keep putting pressure on them," he assured us. "In the meantime, I want to keep you off all foods and liquids, and we're going to keep you on the IV to see if we can get your potassium and iron levels a little higher. I'm increasing your steroid IV dosage and keeping you on the antibiotics to be sure there's no infection. That should help."

Then Dr. York glanced down at my arms. They were blanketed in black and purple bruises from the multiple IV lines they'd had to run when one after another blew a vein. By this point, when I was given any medication or even the saline intravenously, I begged for more pain medication.

"Hmm," he said, holding my right arm up for a closer look. "I think we're going to have to put in a PICC line."

A PICC line? Isn't that what they use to administer the serious drugs or put in for long-term stays? That's when it hit me. I wasn't going home anytime soon.

I had already lost twenty-five pounds, so clearly my body was not getting the nutrition I needed through my GI tract. Dr. York told me that the nurse would get me started on total parenteral nutrition (TPN) right away so that nutrients could be administered directly into my veins. Without the nutrients from the TPN, I couldn't even survive.

Moments later, a doctor in a surgical mask and sterile gown

entered the room, numbed my right arm, made a small incision in the middle of my left bicep, and inserted a long, thin, hollow, flexible tube, which he called a catheter, into the vein. He then gently navigated it up my arm and to the larger veins close to my heart.

"You'll need to be very cautious with this," he cautioned me. "If any bacteria gets in, it could kill you."

I gulped. *Why does every treatment intended to help me seem to have the potential to kill me?*

Every time the nurse came in to change the dressings over the line, all other staff and visitors—including Ryan—had to leave the room. Then she put a mask and a sterile gown on both herself and me. As she worked, I would hold my breath and pray that nothing bad would happen.

On the upside, Dr. York finally won his battle with the insurance company and was able to start me on Entyvio. Between this new medication and having zero food pass through my GI tract, my inflammation levels started coming down. Yet I was coming up on ten days in the hospital with no release date in sight.

Hallmark Christmas movies and old episodes of *Friends* helped pass the time, but I didn't know how much longer I could take this. I wanted to go home. I wanted to see my kids. I wanted to feel healthy again.

One day as I lightly touched the bandage over the PICC line that was pumping nutrients directly into my bloodstream, I could feel the warm flood of tears forming behind my eyes.

God, I need you to pull me out of this, I prayed silently.

Just then the door opened, and one of my nurses poked her head in. "Hi, Danielle," she said, smiling kindly. "How are you doing today?"

I pushed back the tears and tried to sit up without undoing any of the wires.

"Okay, thanks." I smiled back, draping the heart monitor cord over the side of the bed. What I really wanted to say was, *I haven't seen my kids in more than a week, I'm miserable, and I just want to go home*, but I was afraid that if I did, the tears would start flowing.

She glanced at the television screen. *"White Christmas!"* She beamed. "That's one of my favorites." Then she circled around to the other side of the bed and lifted my hand. "You know the drill."

Sadly, I did. Because I was receiving TPN and high doses of steroids, I had to have my blood sugar levels tested every four hours, followed by an insulin shot nearly every time. I was starting to feel like a pin cushion, and my fingertips felt like I had burned them a million times on a hot frying pan.

"There." After pricking my finger, she smiled again. "That wasn't so bad." She then checked my monitors and IV bag. Before she left, she gently touched my shoulder. "Call me if you need anything, okay?"

I smiled and nodded as she left the room. As much as I hated being in the hospital, the staff had been wonderful and so encouraging. They wanted to get me out of there as much as I did.

Alone once again, I settled back into the bed and glanced toward the window. The sun shone brightly into the room. On the sill sat homemade cards my three precious children had created for me.

What are they doing right now? I wondered. *Probably playing with the dog in the backyard.* I smiled at the thought, and the tears came once again.

Ten days. Ten days without seeing or holding my children since they were still recovering from their colds. Ten days of wearing a thin hospital gown and not being able to take a shower. Ten days of doing nothing but channel surf while nurses came and went, poking and prodding me on each visit. At least I finally had enough strength to get out of bed and sit in a chair. *Baby steps*, I told myself. *Baby steps.*

Two days later, on November 17, my kids were finally over their colds and allowed to visit me. I was so excited I could barely stand it. But I was also worried.

"My children are all young," I told Dr. York when he stopped by on his rounds. "I don't want them to be frightened by seeing me hooked up to all of this." I nodded toward the beeping heart monitor and the ominous-looking bags of fluids feeding the PICC line.

He smiled gently. "Okay, I'll have the nurse slow down your TPN and then unhook you from the PICC line, and you can go outside to see them in the courtyard. How does that sound?"

It sounded wonderful.

After the nurse unhooked me, she helped me change out of my hospital gown. I put on my now baggy sweatpants, a shirt, and a long brown sweater. Then I slowly headed down to the courtyard. As soon as I saw their little faces appear above the bushes, tears filled my eyes and the breath rushed from my lungs. I had almost forgotten what it was like to feel this happy. I took each laborious step to meet them in the middle as quickly as my frail and atrophied body would allow.

Both Easton and Kezia ran toward me. Kezia made it into my arms first, followed immediately by Easton.

"Mommy! Mommy!" he chirped excitedly, handing me a little pot with white flowers in it that he proudly informed me he had picked out all by himself.

Asher was slightly more cautious. The poor little guy was still worried that he might get me sick if he got too close. Still, the giant smile he flashed when he tentatively presented me with a little fuzzy garden gnome before retreating to the protection of Ryan's arms sent my heart and spirit soaring.

I stayed with them as long as I could before exhaustion finally got the better of me.

"Okay, guys," Ryan announced, "time to go and let Mom get some rest." Before they left, Ryan took a picture of the four of us on the little bench in the courtyard. When I'd been sick in the past, I rarely allowed photos. I didn't want to have any physical memories of those times. But eventually I realized that looking back at those pictures helps you realize how far you've come when feelings of defeat and hopelessness inevitably creep in. This photo was purposeful. I willed myself to smile so that I could look back on it—in weeks, months, or even a year—and be thankful for the progress I'd made.

Easton, who was sitting on the far end of the bench, reached his arm all the way across Asher and Kezia just so his hand could touch me before Ryan snapped the photo.

If ever there was a time I thought for sure my heart might actually burst, that was it.

———————————

The days that followed were tedious and monotonous. With little else to do, I occasionally poured out my fears with a weak and shaking hand in a journal I'd brought with me to the hospital.

I'm exhausted emotionally and physically. From being poked. Prodded. Shot up. Woken up 3 to 4 times through the night for medications or vital checks. Poked every morning at 6, just as I've fallen back to sleep, for daily blood draws to monitor my inflammation levels, hemoglobin, and a billion other things that my life is clinging to by a thread.

Dwelling on how I felt only made me more despondent, so I flipped through the channels on TV. Nothing interested me. *I suppose I could create our Thanksgiving menu*, I thought. Surely, I would be out of here by then. Why not get a head start? I grabbed a pad of paper and a pen from my nightstand, pulled up the PDF of *Celebrations* on my laptop, and started scrolling.

Brined and roasted turkey with pan gravy, of course, I thought, jotting it down. *No, let's start with the appetizers.* I scratched out the turkey and in its place wrote, "Crab-stuffed mushrooms." *Ooh, yes, that sounds good.* Then I added spinach artichoke dip with veggies and Simple Mills crackers, followed by the turkey, roasted garlic mashed cauliflower, cranberry sauce, green bean casserole with crispy shallots, smoky candied bacon sweet potatoes, and roasted brussels sprouts with bacon jam.

My mouth started to water. *Is this crazy?* I wondered. After all, I had expected to be hospitalized for only three days. It had now been almost two weeks—without any solid foods—and I *still* didn't feel that much better. I turned my head toward the window. The little white flowers from Easton stood tall and bright in the sunrays that filtered in. I glanced at the happy drawings that my children had colored for me and Ryan had placed throughout the room. *No, Danielle*, I scolded myself, *You* will *be home in time for Thanksgiving. And you might even get to eat some of the food.*

The next day the hospital doctor came by to see me. "It looks like we can release you tomorrow."

A huge sigh of relief escaped my lips. The next day was November 20. I was going to be home in time for Thanksgiving after all!

"You'll still have the PICC line," he continued. "A home health nurse will go to your house every couple of days to check on you. But someone will show you and your husband how to hook you up so you can get the TPN every night."

Wait. I'll still have the PICC line? The thought terrified me. *I don't want my kids to see that. And what if something goes wrong with the PICC line?*

He continued giving me instructions, but all I could hear was the warning *If bacteria gets in it, it could kill you* echoing in my head.

After the doctor left and I texted Ryan and a few close friends the good news, I looked around the room that—until now—had felt so stifling. Suddenly it felt safe and comfortable. My mind was racing with doubts and fears. I pulled out my journal and tried to form the concerns shouting in my head into coherent words on the page.

Isolation. Which almost drove me to pull my hair out, but somehow also feels comfortable.

Will home be too much for me? Will the kids and all the chaos overwhelm me? Will they understand that I'm home, but still only 20% myself? That my strength is nonexistent?

I'm afraid to start eating again. It's been 9 days on only ice chips, 15 on liquids. I don't want a setback. Will food hurt?

I looked in the mirror today at my skeletal figure and cried. I barely recognize myself. Will my husband find me horrifying to look at?

The questions continued to come. How was I going to move? Shuffling even five steps down the hospital hallway while pushing my IV pole during my required daily laps still exhausted me. I'd have to climb fifteen stairs just to get into the house. Then another eight or so to get to my bedroom. How was I going to do that? And what would happen if Kezia accidently pulled at my PICC line?

I hadn't realized how genuinely close to death I'd been until I'd talked with Dr. York a few days before. Early in my stay, he had mentioned my albumin (a protein produced in the liver) levels and uttered the words *mortality rate* a few times, but I wasn't lucid enough to understand. I now knew that I had been at a 3 when I was admitted, which was considered nearly normal. After the colonoscopy, my level dropped to 1.4. The level in people experiencing organ failure is around 1.2. It was hard to believe my levels had dropped that quickly. And my hemoglobin (which carries oxygen from the lungs to the body's organs and transports carbon dioxide back to the lungs) had dropped from a 10 at admission, which was already on the low end, to a 6. I was now severely anemic. Clearly, the colonoscopy procedure had sent my system over the cliff.

I started to think about the protein and banana shakes I drank constantly after my flare with Easton and then again with Kezia. *Those shakes may have literally saved my life. My body wasn't just craving protein; it was demanding it to live.* If only I could have tolerated those shakes this go-round, maybe I wouldn't have been in this predicament. My brain continued to process. *That's probably why I also craved baked potatoes with each of my postpartum flares. I thought they were just a neutral food that felt safe to me. But I needed the extra potassium on top of the bananas in the shake. It really is all about food!*

I hated being on the medications; they terrified me. I'd had my first infusion of Entyvio through my PICC line, so what would happen once I was released from the hospital? The thought filled me with hope and terror simultaneously. On the one hand, I'd have to endure infusions every eight weeks. *And it's new,* I reminded myself. They didn't know yet what life would look like for me as a fifty-, sixty-, or seventy-year-old woman. Would I have a weird growth sticking out of my head by then? Or would I spend a lifetime being sick with colds and flus because it suppressed my immune system? Would I be able to snuggle and comfort my sick children as they grew up, or would I have to quarantine myself and leave them to fend for themselves?

On the other hand, if my system responded to the Entyvio, it promised me remission—not just for a year or during a pregnancy, but potentially for years.

I leaned my head back against the pillow and pondered it more seriously. What if it offered me a chance to live day to day not worrying if something I accidentally ate or did—or forgot to eat or do— would send me into a flare? I hadn't realized it until I thought back over the last decade, but while food was warding off symptoms, I was constantly stressed about it. And we had clearly figured out that any type of underlying stress could cause me to flare up. What if this new treatment offered a life where I didn't have to have a fear of certain foods always lingering in the back of my mind? Where I could indulge in a slice of gluten-free pizza or some ice cream once in a while without regretting it immediately, wondering what the consequences would be? Where I could be fully present for my kids? A life where I could finally breathe for a little bit?

My eyes filled with tears. I was so ready for that relief. And yet I'd worked so hard for a decade to avoid this. Ten years ago, Remicade had been the only available option, and back then it involved lengthy infusions. Entyvio had fewer side effects and a shorter infusion time, so I felt grateful that I'd at least bought myself enough time to reap some benefits.

I shook my head to clear it. I had so many questions, and I needed to get some rest before I headed home. *Home. That's what's important here. I'm going home. To Ryan and to our kids. I need to focus on that. To dream about that tonight.*

The next day I awoke bright and early. When the nurse came in to check my vitals, though, she didn't mention anything about my leaving.

"When do you think I'll get released?" I asked. "Later this afternoon, maybe?"

"I'm sorry," she said sympathetically, "you aren't going home today. Your specialist didn't sign off on it."

What?

I immediately reached out to Dr. York's office.

When he came to see me, both his eyes and his tone were filled with genuine remorse. "I'm so sorry, Danielle," he began. "The doctor never should have told you that you were being released. They don't understand how to treat a severe GI case like yours. They just want to push people out the door. I had to fight them tooth and nail on this. You simply aren't ready to go home yet."

Deep down I knew he was right. I was nowhere near 100 percent. I wasn't even at 40 percent. Still, my heart sank at the realization that I would not be giving my babies bedtime kisses that night.

I texted Ryan. Then I texted the friends who'd sent me celebratory messages the day before: "False alarm. Not going home." I typed with no emotion, but when Ryan called a few moments later, I started sobbing. I couldn't help it. I missed the kids so much. Later that morning while Asher was at school, Ryan brought Easton and Kezia by for a surprise visit.

When they walked into my room, I quickly wiped my eyes and put on my biggest and brightest smile. Kezia was wearing a pink tutu with white sparkly leggings and a jean jacket, and as soon as she finished hugging me, she turned on her little toy piano and showed me her new ballet moves. Easton just stared at all the machines. I hated that they had to see me like this, but being able to see, hold, and kiss them both was the best medicine I could have received.

Once again Dr. York allowed me to unhook the PICC line so we could leave the machines behind and go down to the cafeteria. I had called Ryan's mom, Barb, to see if she could pick up some art supplies, which he brought with him. We camped out at a table and did some Thanksgiving crafts and colored for a while. When the nurse came down to check on me, I asked her to bring me a couple of the homemade popsicles I was keeping in the freezer so the kids could have a treat. She happily obliged. I just wanted *something* to feel normal for them—and for me.

After about an hour, Ryan noticed that I was starting to wear down.

"Okay, time to go, guys," he said to the kids.

"Mom?" Easton looked at me expectantly. "Are you coming too?"

"No, sweetie," I said as gently as I could. "Mommy's going to stay here for a little while longer." The disappointment on both their faces was almost too much to bear. Thank goodness Ryan was able to get their things packed up and usher them out of the room before we all started crying. As much as I hated being left behind, the fact that I felt as though I'd run a marathon after just one hour of sitting at a table and coloring proved I wasn't ready to go home yet.

Later that day after school, Asher came separately and, like before, stood at a distance.

"Come give me a hug, Bugs," I said, holding my arms out. But he refused to move, his eyes locked on the PICC line in my arm. My mind raced back to his question before I was admitted to the hospital. *Are you going to die?*

"It's okay, Ash," I said as cheerily as I could. "I'm getting better, and I'm going to be coming home really soon." He didn't budge. I looked him square in the eye. "Bud, Mommy is not going to die. I promise." His lower lip quivering, he came toward me and gave me a hug, careful to avoid touching my left arm. "I love you," I said, gently rubbing his back. "It's going to be okay. Everything's going to be okay."

After Asher left, I couldn't hold back the deluge of tears any longer. As wonderful as it was to see my kids, now that they were gone I felt lonelier than ever. I missed them. I missed Ryan. I missed my parents, my friends . . . my community. I wiped my eyes, reached over for my laptop, and logged on to my Instagram account. *If anyone could understand what I was going through . . .* I began typing:

I'm not going to sugarcoat it. This is hard, y'all. . . . I just have to be honest and say I'm struggling. I'm lonely. I'm bruised and battered. I'm weak. I'm exhausted from being poked and prodded every 4 hours. I miss my family so deeply I feel it in my physical body.

But I'm not without hope. I've recovered from this before. I know I will soon. And I know I'll go home. And I know, somewhere down the line, the God that I believe in will use this trauma to help others. It will not all be in vain.

We've learned more about my body. We've learned where things went wrong, what things went well. We're learning and reevaluating lifestyle, stress, schedules, work. So much is put into perspective when your life hangs by a thread.

It's a lot. But it's good. And I'm going to come out stronger. . . .

You're helping get me through this. And I'm so grateful.

I was full of gratitude. Despite everything, I really was grateful. I didn't understand why I was still struggling. Or why all the tactics that had worked so well before seemed powerless this time around. But just like every other flare, this one had brought with it new lessons. I did understand my body better. And I knew I would emerge from it stronger, with more knowledge to help myself and others feel better and stay healthy.

It's all part of the journey, I reminded myself. *It's all part of the journey.*

17

"Okay, here we are," Ryan said as he pulled into the driveway. It was November 22, 2019, and after I'd spent eighteen days in the hospital, my levels had finally improved enough for Dr. York to remove my PICC line and discharge me. I went home with a cocktail of about twelve different prescriptions that I would need to take for several weeks. Nothing like going from no medicine at all to a dozen heavy-duty drugs—half of them prescribed to combat the side effects caused by the other half.

I inhaled deeply and opened the car door. My legs slowly carried me from the car into the garage, where I was greeted by a large white banner with colorful letters spelling out "WELCOME HOME, MOMMY. WE LOVES YOU" along with scribbles, which I presumed were Kezia's handiwork.

"Go slow, Dani," Ryan said, one hand on my back, the other on my elbow, guiding and supporting me.

I just smiled and laughed. "I don't think there's any other way I *can* go."

I looked up. There they were. Stairs. So *many* stairs. And I was already so unbelievably exhausted. I swallowed hard and willed my right foot to lift me up onto the first stair. Then another. Then another.

Four steps in, three beautiful, precious little faces appeared at the top of the stairway. "Mommy! Mommy!" Easton shouted over and over again as Kezia jumped up and down clapping. Asher, ever the protector, stood right next to her making sure she didn't topple right down into me.

Every fiber of my being wanted to race up those steps, two at a time, to get to those little faces. I wanted to wrap my arms around them and never let go. My legs however, were not quite up to the challenge. *Stay focused on those faces, not on the stairs*, I told myself.

"I'm coming, sister," I said, smiling at Kezia and lifting my foot one more time.

By the time I reached the top, I felt more exhausted than at any time during the previous three weeks. It's amazing how much your muscles atrophy after sitting in bed for so long. But I made it. And talk about a reward! All three of my little angels wrapped their arms around me and hugged me tight. Too exhausted to move and over-whelmed with joy at finally being able to hold my babies again in my own home, I just sat at the top of the stairs hugging them, a smile etched on my tear-stained face. I could practically feel their relief at having me home—especially Asher. He had been so afraid I was going to die. And I could tell from his hug he knew I was still fragile. What a terrible load for a child to bear. I could sense him lighten up a bit when he noticed that all the tubes and wires were gone.

"Okay, everyone," Ryan said, sensing I had reached my energy limit. "Mommy's tired. Let's let her rest awhile, okay?"

"Mommy, I want to dance with you!" Kezia said, holding my hand loosely and twirling around like a ballerina. I so wanted to join her, to pick her up and swing her around in circles while she giggled in delight. But after riding home in the car and tackling the stairs, I was barely able to lift my arms, let alone Kezia.

"Mommy is going to lie down for just a bit," I told her. "But I'll be back out to play with you real soon, okay, sweetie?"

She pouted for a second, but then I leaned over and kissed the tip of her nose. She erupted into giggles.

"What are you laughing about, K-Bits?" Ryan swooped in and lifted her up above his head, making her giggle even harder and distracting her just long enough for me to stand up and slowly make my way toward the bedroom.

My bedroom. Finally. I took a deep breath. The warm, familiar aroma of my autumn essential oil candles filled the air. Ryan must have put them out when he and the kids decorated the house for Thanksgiving. That scent was so much better than the harsh chemical smell of disinfectant that had been stinging my nostrils for the past two weeks. I hoisted myself onto the bed, stunned at how much effort it took.

I ran my fingers along the soft, downy comforter. No more stiff, scratchy hospital sheets that rustled of plastic when I moved or pillowcases that smelled of bleach. I could hear Ryan playing with the kids in the other room, Kezia's sweet laughter a welcome reprieve from the monotonous *click, click, click* of the IV and the incessant beeping of the heart monitor.

Everything in that room reminded me of something or someone I loved—the picture on our nightstand of Ryan and me in Napa right after our wedding, the cards the kids had made for me propped up on the dresser next to Asher's little garden gnome and the little pot of flowers from Easton; my favorite cozy faux-fur blanket—everything was familiar and endearing except . . . *me*.

I barely even recognized the face staring back at me from the mirror on the wall next to my closet. I had wasted away to almost nothing. My ribs and collarbone protruded through my skin, which seemed to hang off my still badly bruised arms. Dark, crescent-shaped circles stood out from under my eyes, my hair was thinning in spots and had lost its natural shine and body, and my skin looked ghastly sallow. I was a far cry from the vibrant, healthy woman on the cover of *Eat What You Love*, which was lying on the chair next to the bed. I could feel a warm flood of tears forming behind my eyes. I was so tired of crying.

Stop it, Danielle, I said to myself, pushing the tears back. *This was just a setback. Another bump in the road. You will get better. You've bounced back before. You can do it again.*

"Dan," Ryan poked his head in the door. "You okay? Is there anything you need?" Easton was literally wrapped around Ryan's left leg, doing a ride along and wearing a big, goofy grin.

I made a funny face, and my little boy immediately burst into peals of laughter. "No, thanks," I said. "I've got everything I need."

———————

For the next few days, when I wasn't having to excuse myself to my room to take an antianxiety pill to combat the incredibly short nerves and patience levels the prednisone was giving me, the kids and I cuddled together on the sofa watching Disney movies nonstop. Disney+ had launched while I was in the hospital, so my first order of business was introducing my kids to all the classics. Kezia's favorites quickly became *Moana* and *Cinderella* (but only the "Bibbidi-Bobbidi-Boo" scene). We watched the old Mickey Mouse Christmas classics, *The Santa Clause* (both 1 and 2), the first two *Home Alone* movies, and any other Christmas movie we could fit in. It was glorious. Just lying on the couch with those three little warm bodies was doing wonders for my recovery. My energy level was still next to nothing, and more than once the kids had to wake me up after I'd fallen asleep twenty minutes into a movie. Still, just being home with my family and eating solid foods made me feel human again.

I was also heartened by friends who called me with their well wishes and was floored when a couple who lived in Maui urged us to visit early in the new year and spend two weeks in their home while they were on the mainland. When I pulled out my journal, I had to acknowledge that even though my prayers hadn't all been answered the way I'd hoped, God wanted me to know that he had never left my side.

> *For the first time in years, I think I can finally feel that God is there. I've been feeling so abandoned and unheard. But there've been 3 moments this week that I just don't think I can chalk up to coincidence. When I really look at them, I can't help but feel like he's trying to show me that he's good and he feels my pain. Even though he's not healing me yet. Or at least not in the way I expect and hope for.*
>
> *I know he's going to use all of this somehow.*

Ryan had surprised me with a thirteen-foot Christmas tree that fit perfectly in our new living room with vaulted ceilings. He, his dad, and the kids decorated the whole house while I lay on the couch and watched. Normally I handle all the holiday decorations because while Ryan loves the finished product, he can't stand dealing with the boxes, clips, and fiddly bits. As much as I hated not being able to do it myself, I was incredibly grateful that in addition to handling all the housework and taking care of the kids and me, he took the time to make the house look special for the holidays.

"It's a good thing Thanksgiving is late this year," he said, hanging the last of the ornaments on the tree. "Otherwise, I don't know how we would have fit all this in."

"I told you I would be home by Thanksgiving," I said, smiling from the sofa. And the best was yet to come.

———————————

The day before Thanksgiving, my mother and mother-in-law showed up on my doorstep armed with all the ingredients to make a hearty, healthy holiday feast, using the list I'd put together during my hospital stay. My mom even brought her own copy of *Celebrations* to cook from.

"You know, you didn't need to bring that," I teased her, "I *do* have a couple of copies here."

"I like all my bookmarks," she said. "Your job, Danielle, is just to sit right here—" she pointed at a chair pulled up to the counter looking into the kitchen—"and direct us. We'll do everything."

The least I could do was cut the loaves of bread into small cubes for the stuffing. And I could do it sitting down, so I talked them into giving me that one small job while they handled the rest.

As the three of us talked, laughed, and reminisced about past Thanksgivings, I felt an overwhelming sense of love and gratitude for all the people in my life who had helped me when I needed it most over the past several weeks. My parents had sat with me during lonely evenings in the hospital and even brought a Christmas wreath to hang on the IV pole so I had something that smelled great and was pretty to look at. My in-laws had helped Ryan with dinner and bedtime nearly every night. Our incredibly selfless and loving childcare provider, Maria, kept the kids happy and as preoccupied as possible during the days while Ryan was at the hospital with me, running Asher to and from school and sports, or working on projects for Against All Grain. Our community of friends chipped in with carpooling or inviting Asher over for playdates. And of course, at the top of my list of people to be thankful for was Ryan.

Throughout my entire UC journey, this man, my high school sweetheart, had been right by my side. He fought for me when I couldn't fight for myself. He never made me feel as though I were a burden. He carried the entire weight and responsibility of our home, our kids, and my business. He also managed my care in the hospital when I was incapable of caring for myself. He sat by my side during the day, leaving only to pick up the kids from school; to bring me gut-healing foods like bone broth, homemade popsicles, or mashed sweet potatoes; or to put the kids to bed—often coming back to be with me after they were asleep and his parents had taken over. He did each of these acts willingly, sacrificially, and without complaint. I didn't always appreciate it, but as exhausted as my disease left me, the truth was, it took an awful lot out of him, too. Still, he led our family tirelessly with strength and grace.

Some statistics show that people with chronic disease have a 75 percent divorce rate—particularly if the wife is the one who is ill. (Our odds would be considered even higher with the loss of a child.) Living with an incurable disease isn't for the faint of heart. It takes passionate courage and tenacity, and we fought every day to let our hardships make us stronger and not tear us apart.

I know Ryan has a greater purpose in life than simply taking care of me. But at the same time, I think God gave him to me because he knew the type of man Ryan was—and that he would fight for me when I couldn't do it for myself.

It's so easy to lose perspective when you're battling a debilitating illness—to forget that there are others around you putting their own problems and difficulties aside so they can be there for you. It takes every ounce of your strength to focus on getting well. But I was so overwhelmingly grateful that so many of them would be sitting around my own dining room table the following evening so I could tell them how much they all meant to me. And I had already started some fun online shopping for Christmas to *show* them how grateful I was.

By the time my mom and Ryan's mom left, our refrigerator was literally packed to the hilt with delectable dishes just waiting to be finished off or reheated the next day. In addition to everything on my list, they had made every other dish in the Thanksgiving chapter of my *Celebrations* cookbook: an eighteen-pound turkey marinating in a brine of pinot grigio, honey, garlic, onions, thyme, allspice, peppercorns, juniper berries, bay leaves, and anise seeds; creamy green bean casserole; velvety garlic mashed cauliflower; savory apple-sausage stuffing; roasted brussels sprouts with bacon jam; herbed drop biscuits; tart cranberry sauce; and my favorites—a creamy spiced maple pumpkin pie and a caramelized coconut sugar custard pie layered with concentric patterns of pecans—for dessert. Ryan's dad had even made a handful of appetizers from the New Year's Eve chapter—including decadent crab-stuffed mushrooms and silky spinach-artichoke dip with crudités.

The next afternoon, about four hours before dinner, they would just have to pat the turkey dry, transfer it to the roasting pan, scatter the vegetables around the pan and inside the cavity, and let it roast until the skin was a perfect crispy brown color and the meat inside succulent and moist. They would then heat up the sides and dessert. And the best part? Every last dish was free of grains, gluten, dairy, and refined sugar. I could eat everything.

"Did you have fun today?" Ryan asked as we settled into bed.

"I did." I smiled up at him. "Your mom and my mom really cooked up a storm!"

"I know! I just looked in the fridge. We're going to be eating leftovers for a month!" he said, laughing.

"That's fine by me," I said. "I probably won't be able to eat too much tomorrow anyway. I'm actually looking forward to nibbling on it all week, especially the pumpkin pie. That always tastes better two or three days later anyway."

"Assuming there's any left," he joked. Then his voice became a little more serious. "You're sure having everyone over here tomorrow isn't going to be too much for you?"

"I'm positive," I assured him. "You have no idea how much I've been looking forward to this."

Truth be told, I was a little worried. Even though I knew our parents would handle the lion's share of the last-minute food prep and hostessing duties, just staying awake and alert through an entire Thanksgiving dinner would push my still-weakened system to the max. And I knew I would want to jump in and help, so I'd have to be told to sit down and relax repeatedly. But there was no way I was going to miss out on this dinner.

Ever since I was a little girl, I'd dreamed of hosting a big holiday gathering with family and friends in my own home, with my own homemade meal. I may not have done the prep work this time, but I had worked long and hard to create every last dish that would be on that table tomorrow. This meal would represent everything I'd accomplished over the past ten years—every hour spent experimenting in the kitchen to get the tastes and textures of the foods I'd always loved just right. It would reflect every bit of research I'd done to discover the difference between almond, coconut, and cashew flour; why bread rises; how to thicken gravy or a green bean casserole sauce without dairy and flour; and which spices and seasonings work best with which protein or vegetable. It was the culmination of every trip to the grocery store or the farmer's market, and the endless hours testing new products or scrolling through online stores to track down the freshest and healthiest ingredients.

I hadn't just been looking forward to this meal since I went into the hospital; I'd been looking forward to it for a lifetime.

———————

The day started as it always does for us at Thanksgiving—with the Macy's Thanksgiving Day Parade on the TV and a blazing fire in the fireplace. We watched the floats go by and enjoyed my favorite part—snippets from the latest Broadway shows—as my mom pulled a steaming batch of my grain-free cinnamon rolls out of the oven, their syrupy cinnamon swirl filling the dough, and iced them with cashew-coconut glaze streaming into the spirals and down the sides. I was so thankful that I had frozen the batch I'd made in early October for an Instagram Live event.

After the parade ended, the kids went outside with Ryan for a game of baseball while his dad, Dwight, pulled the salt-and-herb-infused, brined turkey from the fridge. I sat at the counter and talked him through the final prep so he wouldn't have to read the instructions in the book. It was a little bittersweet not being able to finish it myself, but the trade-off of spending a little extra one-on-one time with Ryan's dad made it all worthwhile.

Eventually, three o'clock rolled around, and virtually everyone I loved—Grandma Marge and Grandpa Wynn, both sets of our parents, and all my kids—had piled into our home. The next day, my sister and her family would be flying in from Denver, and my brother and his family were coming in from the city to enjoy the leftovers.

The kitchen counter was blanketed with every single Thanksgiving dish from my book—all lovingly made by the hands of my family. The turkey skin was perfectly golden and crisp, and I was able to stand long enough to join my dad in our annual tradition of making the gravy together, blitzing the caramelized onions and roasted garlic in the blender with the pan drippings. Then we added a little fresh turkey stock and simmered it all on the stove. As it thickened, Dad added the extra pinches of cracked pepper he always snuck in, and I threw in a sprig of thyme to add more flavor.

Next to the turkey, my cauliflower mash—which I had perfected since my first SCD Thanksgiving—was piled high in billowy mounds in my mom's casserole dish. To its left sat the signature butter-filled mashed potatoes that Ryan loved. It was the only dish I couldn't eat, but at least *this* year, instead of the alternative being a watery mess, the real thing would have some stiff competition!

Grandma Marge, in her signature style, had offered to prepare multiple dishes, but I let her bring only one—my Smoky Candied Bacon Sweet Potatoes—so she could enjoy the evening and finally have a break. Next to that, the stuffing, with its impeccably evenly cut squares of grain-free bread (if I did say so myself), was studded with sausage, apples, celery, mushrooms, and tons of fresh herbs. The aroma of its parsley, sage, rosemary, and thyme filled the kitchen.

Steam was still rising from the green bean casserole, creamy and decadent even without canned cream of mushroom soup and sour cream, as Mom sprinkled freshly fried shallots on top. Ryan's mom drizzled sweet and salty bacon jam over a tray of crispy brussels sprouts that she'd pulled from the oven.

A freshly baked batch of my biscuits were nestled in a basket at the end of the counter, covered by a towel to keep them warm. Alongside them, still-warm-from-the-oven pumpkin and pecan pies—both without refined sugar, dairy, or grains—waited to be enjoyed after the meal.

As I surveyed the scene from my spot on the sofa, it all looked perf—"Ah! I almost forgot the cranberry sauce," I called out to Ryan's mom. "I took it out of the freezer yesterday. It's in a jar down in the garage fridge."

"On my way!" she called back, darting down the stairs.

Silly as it sounds, that cranberry sauce was a huge win for me. My dad had always loved the canned kind that he would cut into discs and pour into a bowl, but I had *finally* won him over from that sugary, gelatinous stuff to my homemade version—boiled fresh cranberries with orange zest and honey. Watching him dig into that tart yet sweet crimson treat was going to be one of the highlights of my day.

The cranberry sauce safely in place on the counter, everyone took turns going through the buffet while I sat on the sofa with a heating pack for my sore and aching back. I had ended up putzing around the kitchen and doing more than I should have, but I'd mostly watched with gratitude. While my family could have simply picked up an easy, store-bought meal, they had honored me by graciously taking it upon themselves to make a dinner from scratch that I could eat and that would nourish all our bodies.

Once everyone took their seats in the dining room, I could hear forks hitting the plates and murmurs of contentment coming from everyone around the table. I smiled as I listened to them congratulating each other on a job well done and exclaiming how wonderful the food tasted. I gingerly lifted myself from the sofa and headed into the kitchen to grab my plate. I stared at all the dishes so lovingly prepared and inhaled the familiar aromas. I knew it wouldn't be wise to load up since I hadn't eaten solids for so long, but I had to have a small spoonful of everything.

Ryan smiled and scooted his chair over to make room for me at the table. With each bite, I thanked God that I was alive, that I wasn't on TPN, and that I was actually able to nibble on some of the food. As I savored each and every morsel, I envisioned the food bringing me health and strength. I celebrated this meal as an opportunity to treat my body with the love and nurturing it deserved. I also celebrated food itself. Not only had it saved me physically, but it had also saved the communal gatherings I loved, those times when I could join my loved ones around the table.

Once I'd eaten as much as my still-recovering system would allow, I froze two full meals to enjoy a couple of months down the road—another landmark to get well for.

———————————

After the last of the relatives had left, the leftover morsels had been neatly wrapped and stored in the fridge or freezer for another day, and the kids were asleep, Ryan and I settled on the sofa, the twinkling lights of the Christmas tree bathing the otherwise darkened room in a warm holiday glow.

"You did great, babe," Ryan said, draping his arm over my shoulder so I could cuddle up against him. "Everybody loved the food."

"Mmm . . ." I sighed contentedly. "Of course, I didn't actually *make* any of it."

"Yes, you did, Dan," Ryan corrected me emphatically. "You may not have done the cutting, pouring, or mixing, but there wasn't a dish on that table that would have existed without you. You *made* that meal happen."

I snuggled up a little closer.

"Something else bothering you?" he gently massaged my aching shoulders and lower back. "You seem a little preoccupied."

He was right. I was distracted. As wonderful as tonight had been, watching everyone enjoy one helping after another of delicious, grain-free, gluten-free, dairy-free food, I just couldn't seem to shake the question that had been buzzing around my mind since this last flare started—*Why hadn't the food been enough?*

"It's just . . ." I searched for the right words. "I *know* food makes a difference. I've seen it. I've experienced it. And I've heard from and met hundreds of thousands of other people over the past decade on the blog and on tour who have seen and experienced it too. So why didn't it work this time?"

"Well . . ." Ryan paused for a second. "Maybe it did."

"Ryan, I was in the hospital for eighteen days. On a PICC line. And now I'm taking a whole cocktail of drugs every day just to get back to normal. Or to mitigate the side effects that come from the other drugs." I paused before adding, "I probably should have died."

"But you didn't," Ryan said. "You were struggling, yes, but it wasn't until the colonoscopy that things *really* went downhill. You can't blame the food for that."

"That's true."

Ryan turned to face me. "Remember that flare you had after Asher was born?"

How could I forget? "Yes," I said, nodding.

"And you were upset because you had just started following the Specific Carbohydrate Diet, but it wasn't working?"

I nodded again.

"What did you learn from that?"

"That every situation is different. Foods and supplements affect people in different ways, and once a flare reaches a certain level, food alone isn't always enough to stop it."

"Right. And after Aila?" he asked gently.

My throat constricted a little, and I felt that familiar stinging in my nose every time I heard her name. "I realized that things like stress, hormonal changes, and grief can bring on flares and make them worse."

"And after Easton?"

I thought about the media events and book promotions Ryan had suggested I bow out of, and the special supplements and oats I ate so I could breastfeed longer. "That I need to slow down and listen to what my body is telling me. I can't always put everyone else's needs and health before my own."

"What have you learned about medicine?"

"That even with a proper diet, sometimes it *is* necessary," I admitted dejectedly.

"But . . ." he nudged me, his mouth curving into a slow, encouraging grin.

"That doesn't mean food doesn't work or I'm a failure."

"Exactly." He took both my hands in his. "Dani, look at everything you've done in the past ten years—everything you've put your body through. You've experienced five pregnancies; suffered two horrific losses; delivered three beautiful, healthy children—all by cesarean and all requiring a full run of antibiotics, which you *know* wipe out your system. You've nursed babies, lost sleep, moved homes multiple times, run a business and managed employees, and written four cookbooks. And you've gone on four grueling, nationwide book tours and a bus tour where you barely slept. You've done all this while trying to manage a severe autoimmune disease *and* be a full-time wife and mom! You've been burning the candle at both ends and in the middle for the last ten years without a single break. Babe, that'd be enough to tax *anyone's* system, let alone one as compromised as yours. Who's to say this last flare wasn't just your body's way of telling you, enough!"

Wow. I hadn't thought about it that way.

"So," he said cheerily, "how about if instead of beating yourself up, we focus on the all the amazing things you and food *have* accomplished?"

———————————

Later that night, while Ryan started a few long-overdue loads of laundry, I took advantage of the extra pillows and propped myself up in bed with my recipe journals and a notepad. As near as I could tell, I'd developed close to 1,200 recipes, each of which was featured either on the blog, in one of my cookbooks, or both. Plus I had a handful of others that were still "in the works." Like my mom's shepherd's pie, which now that I had figured out the cream of mushroom soup piece, was almost ready to go. *Still haven't figured out the mac and cheese*, I quietly berated myself. But still, Ryan was right. That record *was* something to be proud of!

I was even prouder of something else. I pulled out the small stack of thank-you letters and cards I kept tucked away in the back of my recipe journal. They were some of my favorites, and I would go back and reread them whenever I was discouraged or needed a reminder that I wasn't alone in this.

My mind suddenly flashed to the little activity I had done with the kids this morning before everyone arrived at the house. I flipped the page of my notepad over.

"This Thanksgiving," I scribbled, "I am thankful for . . . my community. I am thankful for their support, their understanding, their encouragement, and the constant reminder that what I am doing every day in my kitchen is making a difference, not just for my health, but for the health of countless other people suffering just like me."

I thought for a second before starting to write again. "I am also thankful for food and its power not only to nourish but to heal our bodies."

"What are you doing?" Ryan asked, walking into the room.

"Just making a list of things I'm thankful for." I smiled.

"I hope I'm on there!" he said, laughing.

"Oh, don't worry," I teased, "you're definitely on here!"

"Well, don't wear yourself out," he cautioned, sitting down on the edge of the bed and pulling off his shoes. "You look tired."

"You're right." I hated to admit it, but I was. I had forgotten how exhausting writing could be. "I just want to finish this."

He nodded toward the nightstand. "Why don't you use your laptop? You said it's easier, right?"

"That's a good idea," I agreed. I had been meaning to check Instagram anyway to see if anyone had run into problems with any of the Thanksgiving recipes. I logged on to the site and typed in #celebrationscookbook.

"Ryan," my voice cracked. "Look."

He slid over to my side of the bed and turned the screen ever so slightly. "What is that . . . brussels sprouts?" he asked.

"Yes," I said, tears cascading down my cheeks. Photos of the same dishes that had just graced my kitchen countertops appeared in little squares on my screen. In addition to the roasted brussels sprouts with bacon jam, I saw images of spinach artichoke dip and green bean casserole; candied bacon sweet potatoes, garlic mashed cauliflower, pumpkin pie with its signature golden custard and leaf cutouts donning the top, and herbed drop biscuits. I scrolled through photo after photo—thousands of them—showcasing the dishes people had made from *my* cookbook to celebrate their special day.

"Why are you crying?" he asked.

I wiped the tears from my cheeks. "There are probably a billion Thanksgiving recipes out there, but all these people trusted me enough to serve *mine* to their families—on the biggest food holiday of the year!"

"Well, that's awesome, Dani," he said, smiling. "See? I told you. Your food is fantastic." He leaned in and kissed me. "You *are* making a difference, Danielle. And your food is helping save people in more ways than just by improving their health. Don't you ever forget that."

Epilogue

In those first few weeks home, I struggled to go back on an extremely restricted diet. The first few times I tried to eat bone broth, I gagged. It reminded me too much of the hospital and couldn't satisfy my hunger. Pretty much anything that I knew I was supposed to eat made me nauseated, and I was continuing to lose too much weight too quickly. I just needed to get whatever I could into my body to try to get enough calories. That looked like six slices of toasted Udi's gluten-free bread, an Orgain protein shake, and sheep's milk yogurt for nearly every meal. Or at 2 a.m., when the prednisone kept me awake and made me famished.

I had thought the new medication would allow me to relax a bit around food. I hadn't planned on going crazy, but I had been looking forward to eating store-bought, gluten-free baked goods once in a while and not having the constant fear that something would cause a flare-up. But even after my sixth infusion of Entyvio (while still on the prednisone), my health hadn't improved. I was still in what my doctor considered a flare-up. I had always bounced back fairly quickly from them in the past, and I had to attribute this prolonged setback to depending a little too heavily on the medications and easing up a bit too much on my diet.

So early in the new year, I reminded myself of what my body had needed to heal in the past. As the weeks passed, I couldn't deny that I *did* notice a big difference in my day-to-day symptoms when I controlled what I ate. It was a good reminder that, to get into full remission, I needed to take to heart everything I'd learned over the past ten years.

By the middle of February 2020, I was stronger and had more energy than I'd had since the previous October. I could walk two miles, albeit slowly, whereas at Christmastime I had barely managed to climb the stairs. I was able to wean myself off most of the medications Dr. York had sent me home from the hospital with. I also focused on eating those foods that would help calm the remaining inflammation. The last major medication was the prednisone, and Dr. York didn't want to take me off of it until he was sure the Entyvio was working and I was in remission. Which was not yet apparent. If I ever expected to get off the prednisone, I would need to supplement the anti-inflammatory effects with the food I was eating. And I desperately wanted to get off that drug.

Fortunately, my system was back up and functioning at around 80 percent just in time for us to board a plane and head to Maui to take our friends up on their offer. I knew, even while I was still in the hospital, that my kids were going to need some time to reconnect with me and have my undivided attention in order to heal from the trauma of seeing me in the state I had been in. That's what this trip was about. And as a bonus, we would celebrate my thirty-fifth birthday together as a family in paradise.

It was amazing—thirteen days of uninterrupted family time. No

work, no sports, no school, no errands, no laundry. No hospitals. No obsessing over treatments. Just swimming, napping, exploring, reading, snuggling. And, of course, lots of eating.

Getting a break from all the demands and responsibilities of life was a gift. But it also made me realize that being kind to our bodies is more than focusing on what we feed it; it also involves what we make it do.

"You know how hard these last several months have been," I said to Ryan one morning as we walked along the beach. "I've been thinking about everything you said on Thanksgiving. And whenever I'm reminded of something difficult that's happened in our lives since my diagnosis, I allow myself to sit with that memory. You know what? I've come to realize that there's something besides food that has a healing quality to it."

"What's that?" he asked.

"Rest. I think we don't take rest seriously enough."

"I agree," he said.

I stopped walking and looked at him. "I think I need to take the rest of this year off."

His eyebrows shot up in surprise. "Seriously?"

"Yeah," I nodded. "No traveling, no special events, just you, me, and the kids—spending quality time together at home as a family. What do you think?"

He smiled down at me tenderly. "I think it's an excellent idea."

We walked a little farther down the beach.

"You really think you can do it?" he asked, a sly smile on his face. "Not go anywhere or do anything for a whole year?"

"Well . . ." I hedged. "I'll still do *some* things."

"Like?" he asked.

"I do have that memoir to finish. And I can't wait to start cooking again." I smiled. "And baking."

"More?" he asked incredulously. "Dani, you've already created enough recipes to last a lifetime! What's left?"

I thought about that for a moment. "I *still* haven't nailed that macaroni and cheese."

Ryan laughed and swung my hand higher in the air. "Well, if anyone can do it, Danielle, it's you."

Another Note from Me to You

Okay, we're friends now, right? After all, I just bared my soul and told you about my most raw moments. I think that means I can call us friends.

So, friend—you've read this entire book. That leads me to believe that you and I have a lot in common, regardless of which disease or ailment we struggle with and no matter whether or whom we believe in as a higher power.

After being diagnosed with my disease, I spent a lot of time asking, *Why me?* I've come to terms with the fact that I may never fully understand the answer here on earth, but I have been blessed to see my suffering used to help others, which is something I never expected. Though it doesn't take away the pain, it somehow makes it feel worth it.

Do I wish I never had this disease? Of course. Would I trade having my health in exchange for all the good that has come from it? I'm not sure. Food saved me in more ways than one. Yes—it saved my body. But it also saved my dreams. My ideals. It may have saved my marriage. My life as a mom. My hopes of hospitality. Food gave me a career. One could even say food saved my faith.

After Aila passed away, God and I weren't on the best terms.

When I was on the road with my friends Annie and Angie, doing the church tour, I was genuinely inspired by their passion and love for Jesus. I wanted to get back to that place in my own life. I just didn't know how. I hadn't really prayed in almost five years, so talking to God felt like one of those awkward conversations you have with an ex-boyfriend or a once-close friend with whom you've had a falling out.

I was just starting to regain my footing with God when, midway through that tour, my health started declining rapidly. The three of us prayed on the bus every night that God would heal my body. People had "laid hands on me" or "claimed healing over me" countless times before, and I believed it every time, only to wind up feeling like a sucker who had fallen for a two-bit con artist. And each time I experienced a new disappointment, I became more distrustful and skeptical of God.

But one night Annie prayed so passionately, she nearly convinced me that her prayers were going to work. My own prayers didn't seem strong enough. In fact, I wasn't entirely sure I believed they would even be heard. It was the same feeling I'd had in Uganda and after losing Aila all over again. But hers . . . hers were delivered like she and God were on a close enough level that she could look him in the eye and almost demand he do something for me.

I went to bed convinced I would wake up with a new body. That I would wake up free from pain and bleeding, and full of energy and strength.

But then I just got worse.

My faith continued to dwindle after the tour; during those long, lonely days in the hospital; and more so when I got home. Four months later, following those six Entyvio infusions, I was still in what my doctors would consider a flare-up.

My gastroenterologist was beginning to wonder whether that infusion drug was right for me after all and thought I needed something even stronger. At that point, my faith practically hit rock bottom.

Then I started writing this book. And as I reflected on the past decade (and seriously considered scrapping the entire book, or at least the title), I started to realize that maybe God had been there the entire time.

He was there in the gift of the first-class seat I was given on the trip to Uganda; in the mysterious worship music Ryan and I heard in that little makeshift hospital; in a kind British doctor who introduced me to the concept of gut health and the importance of the microbiome; in a compassionate neighbor who reassured me that I was not alone and introduced me to the Specific Carbohydrate Diet; in an unexpected call from a publisher when I was just a stay-at-home mom and self-trained cook; in a blog and a series of *NYT* bestselling cookbooks that have helped thousands of others thrive in the midst of their own health crises; in the restoration of my love (and need) for entertaining; in four beautiful children; in a wonderful, caring husband without whom none of these things would have been possible; and of course, in the fact that I'm still here, alive, learning, cooking, sharing, and growing. (I'm also pretty sure God was there on the beach when I declared that 2020 would be a down year—seriously, who knew?)

I still have doubts and questions. So many questions. But one thing I know for certain is that food has saved my life. God created it, he put just the right people in my path at just the right times to show me how to unleash the power of it, and he has used my journey with it to help others. God may not have answered my prayers the way I had hoped, but he *did* answer them.

If I hadn't gone through everything I did, this book wouldn't exist and you wouldn't be reading it right now, hopefully ready to take what may be *your* first step into the wonderful, life-giving world of grain-free, gluten-free, and dairy-free living, and to discover for yourself the incredible healing power of food.

I hope you'll take that first step. The journey might not always be easy. But I can promise you it will be worth it.

Eat well and feel great, friend.

A Special Note to Caregivers

From Ryan

Hi, I'm Ryan Walker. Because you're reading this, I'm guessing there's someone in your life who is learning to cope with a chronic health issue. Believe me, I know how challenging that can be. When my wife, Danielle, was first diagnosed with severe ulcerative colitis shortly after we were married, my initial response was, "Okay, let's fix this." I quickly discovered it's not that easy. Chronic illnesses can be extremely difficult to deal with, physically and emotionally, both for the patient and those around them. But a little over a decade later, I can promise you that there is no greater or more rewarding investment you can make than in the health and well-being of your loved one.

I know I may come across as extremely empathetic in this book, but believe me, I didn't start out that way. Our journey has taught me a lot about what it means to be a husband, a father, a support system, a caregiver, and an advocate. You, too, are a critical and irreplaceable partner to your loved one, so I'd like to pass along to you some of what I've learned.

- **Don't judge.** One of the most frustrating aspects of auto-immune diseases like ulcerative colitis, Crohn's, and celiac is that they are often misunderstood and, as a result, down-played. People think, *Oh, so you can't eat bread*. No big deal, right? Wrong. Chronic autoimmune diseases are never resolved by simply eliminating a single food from your diet. They're far more complicated than that. Even the medical community can't agree on the best course of treatment.

Danielle and I have spent years navigating a delicate bal-ance between diet, supplements, medicine, and self-care (i.e., eliminating stress, getting enough sleep, etc.) and even then, a flare-up can quickly escalate into a life-or-death situation. Ten years ago, when Danielle came to me in tears because of the pain she was experiencing, my knee-jerk reaction would likely have been, *It's all in your head*. Believe me, it's not. As a caregiver, one of the most important things you can do for your spouse or loved one is to take their situation seriously, honor their experience, and respect their pain.

· **Communicate.** Another challenge many couples face when dealing with a chronic illness is not wanting to burden their spouse with their problems . . . until it's too late. One of the reasons I married Danielle is that she is a very strong, smart, independent woman, and if there is one thing she *never* wants to be, it's a burden. Unfortunately, sometimes she hides her symptoms from me, and I don't realize there's a problem until things have spiraled out of control. Likewise, I have a tendency to put on a brave face, thinking I always have to be strong so she won't worry. Trust me, neither approach ever ends well.

A number of years ago, Danielle was really struggling. She was too weak to even get out of bed, leaving me to take care of her; our one-year-old son, Asher; the dog; the laundry; the house—everything—all while working a full-time job. I remember sitting down on the stairs by myself—completely overwhelmed—and just sobbing. Meanwhile, a few feet away, Danielle was doing the same thing. You need to approach chronic illness as a team and keep the lines of communication open. You're not helping anyone by trying to go it alone or taking on more than you can handle. Lean into one another. Be collaborative. Tell each other how you're feeling. And remember, it's okay to say, "I'm not okay today."

· **Be an advocate.** As important as two-way communication is, there will be times when your loved one is going to need you to speak on their behalf—especially when dealing with the medical community. Danielle is a strong-willed and independent woman, but when she's sick, she's so physically and emotionally wiped out that she doesn't always have the wherewithal to follow everything that's being said (often very quickly and with a lot of medical jargon), to ask questions, or to describe her symptoms fully and accurately. My job—and yours—is to serve as a proxy.

Keep a detailed list of symptoms, irregularities, medications, dates, and everything else that can help the doctors determine the best course of action. Pay attention, take notes, and be prepared to ask the follow-up questions your spouse is too overwhelmed to think of. Also, don't be afraid to challenge the doctor's assumptions. It's okay to ask, "Why are we doing this?" or "Why would we not try that?" Danielle and I learned the hard way that doctors are not always as forthcoming as you'd like them to be. Most are perfectly happy to answer questions when asked, but they're not always inclined to bring things up if you don't press a little.

You may also need to follow up at home, making sure that medications are taken at the right time and your loved one is getting enough rest, eating what they should, not eating what they shouldn't, exercising regularly, and staying on top of all their appointments. That doesn't mean telling them what to do (which never ends well)—it just means giving them a gentle nudge or reminder to take care of themselves. As good as Danielle is about sticking to her diet, there are still times I have to say, "Are you *sure* you should be eating that?" Danielle doesn't get offended or upset. If anything, she's grateful that I'm tracking with her and that I love her enough to make sure she stays healthy.

· **Step up when needed.** Danielle is an amazing wife and mom, but when she goes down with a flare, she goes down hard and often can't even muster the strength to get out of bed, sometimes for days. That's my cue to step it up. Parenting duties we usually share—getting the kids up, dressed, fed, off to school; helping with homework, playtime, bath time, bedtime—all shift to me, as does doing the laundry, making the meals, washing the dishes . . . all of it. And you know what? That's exactly what needs to happen.

When your spouse is sick, the only thing they should be focusing on is getting themselves better. Your job is to take everything off their plate so they can do just that. Eliminate as much stress as you can, help the kids understand that "Mommy needs her rest," and make sure she knows it's okay to ask you for help. Whatever you do, don't make your spouse feel as though they're a burden. They already feel bad enough. The only vibes they should be getting from you when they're down for the count are love and support.

· **Find a support system.** With most autoimmune diseases, there will be stretches of time—sometimes weeks, sometimes months, and sometimes years—when everything runs smoothly. But the potential for a flare-up is always there. And when it hits, it hits hard and often without warning. When that happens, you're going to need help—especially if you have kids. That said, if you don't have a solid support system of friends and family you can turn to in times of crisis, start developing one. I can't tell you how many times I have had to ask my parents to look after the kids so I could take Danielle to the emergency room or sit with her in the hospital, or have asked someone else to sit with her so I could run errands and take care of the kids. Fortunately, we have a lot of family in the area, but if you don't, cultivating a solid network of friends who are aware of your situation and are willing and able to step in if needed can make a world of difference.

· **Accept help when it's offered.** Speaking of your support system, it's okay to ask for and to accept help when it's offered. It's tempting to play the superhero and say, "I've got this," but trying to be a full-time caregiver, parent, and advocate—*and* work a full-time job—can push even the most capable person to the limit. When Danielle was in the hospital, people would often bring meals to the house so I wouldn't have to cook, or they'd volunteer to take Asher for the afternoon so I could have some time to myself. Not only was that very much appreciated, but it made them feel good to be able to help. Remember, you're in this for the long haul. You're going to need a break every once in a while, so when someone offers you one, take it!

· **Take time for yourself.** There's an old proverb that says, "A chain is only as strong as its weakest link." Danielle and I are a team, and I can't be of any use to her if I'm falling apart myself. That said, it's important to make time for yourself so you don't burn out.

Even if it's only thirty minutes a day, giving yourself a little space to breathe, refocus, and recharge can do you a world of good. Also, because autoimmune diseases can be wildly unpredictable, it helps if you can be flexible and even a little opportunistic. One of the reasons I took up running was that it was something I could do at a moment's notice. I didn't have to drive to the gym. I could just grab my shoes and go, allowing me to work some much-needed "me" time into the natural ebb and flow of our situation. Take advantage of that support network you're building and get away for a little while, whether to take a brisk walk around the block while your parents pick the kids up from school, to shoot hoops out in the driveway while someone else prepares dinner, or to slip off to watch a game on TV while your spouse rests. Don't let your role as a caregiver become so all-encompassing that you forget to take care of yourself.

- **Keep an open mind.** Without question, one of the easiest yet most impactful things I did for Danielle was to offer to eat the same way she did. Not only did it save her from having to make two separate meals three times a day, it also eliminated the temptation (and torture) of having all the things she *couldn't* eat within arm's reach. More important, however, it sent the message that she wasn't alone. We were in this together. And I think that meant more to her than anything.

I realize the thought of completely changing the way you eat can be a little daunting and may even feel a little extreme, but my advice to you is this—just give it thirty days. Try some of the recipes in one of Danielle's cookbooks or on her blog. It's not going to hurt anything. And honestly, the food is fantastic. (I personally recommend starting with the short ribs, the Real-Deal Chocolate-Chip Cookies, and—strange as it may sound—the taco seasoning mix.) Does the food taste a little different? Initially, yes, but you won't notice it at the end because it's also great (seriously, the short ribs). And I'm willing to wager that if and when you do go back to the old food, you'll realize, *Oh, I don't really like that anymore.*

Is eating healthy more expensive? Initially, yes. But don't let those first few grocery receipts frighten you. What we've spent restocking our pantry with gut-healthy foods pales in comparison to what we've paid in medical bills over the years. Frankly, given the potential benefits to your loved one's health, not to mention your own, at the end of the day, *not* trying is the bigger mistake.

· **Be patient.** Obviously we believe food has the power to help manage Danielle's autoimmune disease, but food is just one piece of the puzzle. Supplements, exercise, rest, stress reduction, and (at times) medication also play important roles. But it has taken us years to figure out the right combination for Danielle's system. Everybody is different because every *body* is different. What works for one person might not work for another. There is no one-size-fits-all approach. Some things might help a little; others might not help at all.

It may take a lot of trial and error before you figure out what's right for you, so be patient. You aren't going to see results overnight. Remember, you're helping someone make a major lifestyle change. Just like the food, try to give every new protocol thirty days to see if it works. Create a symptom tracker to keep a record of how your loved one feels before, during, and after each addition, elimination, or alteration. It may take a while, but eventually you'll get there.

And whatever you do . . .

· **Never give up.** Danielle and I have been on this journey together for over a decade now. It hasn't always been easy. We've definitely had our fair share of frustrations and disagreements, but looking back, I honestly believe we're better for our experience. We've both had to make sacrifices along the way, and I have no doubt there will be more to come. When you live with someone who is battling an autoimmune disease, you live with the constant fear that something could go wrong at any minute, because it can. Autoimmune diseases don't follow a schedule. They don't care whether you have concert tickets, vacation plans, work commitments, or family coming over for the holidays. Looking back, we know that Danielle's first telltale symptoms started on our wedding day. So savor the good times.

Keep a sense of humor and a positive attitude during the bad times. Communicate. Advocate. Lean on your support system. Ask for help. Be willing to step up when necessary, but also make sure you set aside some time for yourself. Be patient, and try not to let things like broken plans, lack of sleep or money, or the fear of having to give up your favorite deep-dish pizza distract you from what's really important—each other. Because when all is said and done, the health and well-being of your spouse or loved one outweigh every inconvenience, every sleepless night, and every sacrifice.

Ours may not be the life we envisioned for ourselves. No family wants to deal with a chronic illness. But it is an amazing life. And despite all the challenges, Danielle and I wouldn't trade what we have now for anything.

Your journey won't always be easy. Yes, the learning curve is steep. But if you stick with it, I promise that before you know it, it will become second nature. Just know that the love you have for each other makes it all worthwhile. Remember, too, that you're not alone. Millions of people are dealing with the same fears and frustrations that you have. Danielle and I hear from them every day on her blog. In many ways, they've become like our extended family. And they can become yours as well. We're all in this together. And frankly, we're all still figuring it out. But we've made it this far, and we're still going strong. You know what? So will you.

Okay, Danielle, You've Got My Attention. Now . . .

How Do I Get Started?

First things first—good for you! Way to take an active role in your health! Second—you're in luck. Back when I first started reexamining the way I ate, very few people were talking about using food to treat autoimmune disorders. As a result, gut-healthy recipes were hard to come by and usually were not very tasty. (Remember the runny cauliflower soup?) Today, however, there are a ton of options— online, in the supermarket, and even at restaurants. You just have to know what you're looking for. To help you out, I've included a few simple starter lists as well as a handful of my favorite recipes. And that's just the tip of the iceberg. There are *a lot* more where that came from in my cookbooks and at daniellewalker.com. But before you go there, let me see if I can answer a few FAQs to help get you started out on the right foot.

Can I just do exactly what you did?

Probably not. Remember, this kind of lifestyle isn't a quick fix or a one-size-fits-all approach (which my story makes pretty clear!). Everybody's situation is different because *every body* is different. The key is figuring out what foods (and supplements) work for you.

As a general rule of thumb, you want to avoid as many processed and refined foods as possible. The way most of us eat is inherently inflammatory, so the fewer prepackaged convenience foods you eat, the better. (I give a good rundown of things you want to avoid in chapter 9.)

Beyond that, I'd strongly encourage you (with the assistance of a professional naturopathic doctor, if possible) to try an elimination diet. That means no grains or gluten, dairy, legumes, eggs, refined sugar, or processed foods for four weeks so your body can start to heal and you can pinpoint your trigger foods. It'll also help reduce whatever inflammation you're currently experiencing. Then you can slowly reintroduce one new food item every five to seven days to see how your body reacts.

I would also strongly encourage you to keep a food journal, taking note of each specific food and ingredient that causes you pain or discomfort. This is critical! Do not skip this step! This is your baseline and your road map moving forward. You'll want to keep a running log of every single thing you put in your mouth during the day (even if it's just a bite of something your kids left behind on their plate) in one column, and in another, keep track of your symptoms, day by day—or even hour by hour if they're severe. This will not only help you be more mindful of what you're nibbling or snacking on during the day, it will also help you correlate specific symptoms to what you're eating. Once you figure out which foods trigger your symptoms and which ones are safe, you can tailor your meals to fit your specific needs.

That sounds pretty intense. Can I just start slowly? Maybe a couple of days a week?

Again, probably not. You have to commit to this approach or it's not going to work. If you eat a baguette fresh from the bakery on Monday and then make a grain-free loaf of bread on Wednesday, that loaf isn't going to taste anywhere near as good. That's not because grain-free bread isn't delicious (because, believe me, it is!). It's just that your brain will still have fresh memories of that baguette's flavor and texture, and it will still crave it. It takes your body a good thirty days to work through those preferences, so you can't "on-again, off-again" it. In addition, if you keep flip-flopping back and forth, you won't be giving your body enough time to heal, so you will not see the results you are hoping for.

Remember, you have an emotional and mental connection to food, so it can be a little overwhelming to think about shifting everything all at once. It's okay to grieve what you're "losing" through this process. I grieved a lot! You just need to focus on what you're gaining: Health. Energy. Stamina. And joy!

You mentioned a lot of specialty items and ingredients in your book. What if I live in an area where I can't get them, or they're way beyond my budget?

I hear this from a lot of people. This is where the internet can be a godsend. You can find pretty much everything I use in my recipes online. And if it's an ingredient that shows up in a lot of recipes (like almond flour, cashews, or coconut sugar), look for bulk pricing. Most online vendors offer even deeper discounts when you buy in higher volumes. And bear in mind, these foods aren't available only at specialty health-food stores. Walmart, Target, Costco, Sam's Club, and Aldi all carry a wide array of health foods, often at the lowest prices. Thrive Market is also a wonderful online resource for healthy foods at big-box retailer pricing.

When shopping for poultry or meat, you can save money by buying the whole bird or sizable cuts of meat. See if you can find a few friends to go in with you on a side of beef. And don't let any of it go to waste. If you buy a whole chicken, for example, you can roast those two breasts, two thighs and legs, and other dark underside meat for your main course, use the bones for stock, and throw whatever's left into soups or salads. And if grass-fed meats aren't within your budget, don't worry. You are already eliminating additives and potential toxins simply by following a real-foods diet (i.e., meat, fruit, nuts, and vegetables) and avoiding processed foods.

If you can't afford to buy only organic produce, consult the Environmental Working Group's "Dirty Dozen" table at ewg.org to see when buying organic fruits and vegetables makes the most sense. If it's within your budget, it's best to buy organic strawberries, apples, grapes/raisins, celery, peaches, spinach, bell peppers, nectarines, cucumbers, cherry tomatoes, hot peppers, kale, and collard greens.

Some fruits and veggies—like avocados, pineapple, cabbage, sweet peas, onions, asparagus, mangoes, papaya, kiwi, eggplant, grapefruit, cantaloupe, cauliflower, sweet potatoes, and mushrooms—aren't typically sprayed or treated with pesticides, so those should be safe year-round.

You can also save money by buying whole vegetables and fruits rather than precut produce that comes with a premium price. Shopping for seasonal produce will save you money as well. Be sure to stock up on and freeze those seasonal items so you can enjoy them later, too. And always try to buy local produce from your farmer's market or through a community-supported agriculture (CSA) source if possible. Conventional produce from local growers will always be better for you than store-bought fruits and vegetables.

I'm really worried that I'm not going to like the way this new kind of food tastes. Will I eventually get used to it?

I hear you. That was my fear as well. I felt like I was being asked to eat bland, flavorless food that tasted like cardboard (again, the runny cauliflower soup). I wanted to be able to indulge in all the same great tastes and textures I loved growing up but without the guilt—that's why I started creating my own recipes. I'll be honest, some recipes won't taste exactly like the "original," but that doesn't mean they won't be just as tasty. My first attempt at making a healthy chicken Parmesan while following Mad may not have been what I was used to, but it sure did the trick for my comfort food craving. Remember, *different* doesn't necessarily mean *bad*. Once you make the switch and your palate adjusts to the natural goodness of real foods, you won't miss the old stuff at all.

I'd really like to try eating this way, but my spouse and kids aren't as excited about it as I am. How can I get them on board?

That's a tough one. Some people just won't get it—especially if they're healthy and have no driving motivation to change the way they eat. They may even try to tempt you by insisting that you "just try one bite" or argue that changing the way you eat won't make any difference.

You can quote statistics and facts about healthy eating all day, but until they see how good it can be for themselves, it will be a tough sell. But believe me, as soon as your family realizes how good healthy foods can actually taste, they'll likely get on board.

Many years ago, I put together a Thanksgiving PDF of recipes that are almost all now in my *Celebrations* cookbook. I tested all the recipes on my family, and they loved them. But what really helped them make the switch was how they felt after eating our huge meal. They told me (with a note of surprise, I might add), "Normally I eat Thanksgiving dinner and want to lie on the couch for three hours afterward. This tasted amazing, but I'm also not exhausted."

Start slowly, by swapping homemade items for those you buy. For example, make chocolate chip cookies (see page 307 for my recipe) rather than buying the dough at the store. And if they love the ones you made, just stop buying the store-bought kind. Introducing new recipes that taste good always works better than sitting your family down and announcing, "Guess what? We're never buying any of this again. And you're now eating this way."

Children, especially, need to feel ownership over the change, and cannot just be forced to make it. If your kids are used to eating white pasta, you can't suddenly serve them spaghetti squash and *not* expect them to exclaim, "Eww. What is this?" Start by easing them into different foods—maybe make one or two meals a week in which you introduce something that's grain-free or dairy-free and that actually tastes good. Or try mixing rice with cauliflower rice to start.

Most important, when you serve something new, don't say, "Hey, this is gluten-free, dairy-free, legume-free, refined sugar-free, and free of anything else that used to give you joy." As soon as we hear those types of disclaimers, we automatically convince ourselves that we are not going to like it. Instead, let the food be the star. Then, after people have thoroughly enjoyed the meal, you can drop the "-free" bombs and sit back to watch the surprised expressions.

Even if you aren't successful at getting others in your household on board, remember that ultimately *you* are the person you're trying to help. You need to do it for yourself . . . and for them. Go slow, be patient, and don't give up! I promise, after you see how great you start to feel, it will be a little bit easier. And then maybe your spouse will see that it's working and support you.

And just in case your spouse needs a little extra nudge, I asked my husband, Ryan, to write "A Special Note to Caregivers" (see page 279) to help them get on board.

It's one thing to eat this way at home, but what about getting together with friends or extended family, especially during the holidays?

When I first started eating this way, I wondered if I would ever be able to eat out with friends again. The key is to not make a big deal about it. Find out from the host or hostess ahead of time what you can contribute to the meal, then bring something you can eat and others can enjoy along with you.

Or better yet, invite them to your home! Treat your friends and family to a wonderful evening of fun and great, healthy food. My cookbooks and blog are full of friend-and-family-tested-and-approved options that will not only impress your guests, but will introduce them to another way of eating they may never have considered. That's what gathering around the table is all about. Great food should bring us together, not keep us apart, and healthy food *is* great food.

This all feels so overwhelming. Is there anywhere I can turn for extra help and support?

Listen, I get it. I know what it's like to feel sick and exhausted all the time. I know what it's like trying to deal with the side effects of steroids and the toll they take on your body and your self-image. And on top of everything else, now you have a completely different lifestyle to adjust to. It's a lot.

But know this—you are not alone. There are millions of other people out there dealing with chronic health issues—myself included—and we *all* get it. You're not a hypochondriac. It's not all in your head. What you're dealing with is real. And it's hard. But it's also manageable. Yes, there will be bad times. But there will also be good times. Great times, in fact—a lot of them. And the sooner you start taking control of your health, the better you'll feel.

Food has amazing power to heal. Hopefully, my story and all the other testimonials I have shared in this book have convinced you of that. But it's not just about eating healthy. It's also about getting enough sleep and managing your stress level. Stress and anxiety are both massive triggers for flare-ups. Believe me, I learned that the hard way.

It's perfectly normal to feel a little down from time to time. What you're going through isn't easy. Don't try to do it alone. Talk to your spouse, your parents, your siblings, your close friends. Tell them what you need. I think you'll find everyone genuinely *wants* to help. They just might not know how.

There's also a tremendous support network available on my blog at daniellewalker.com/. If you don't know where else to start, start there. The community of encouragers you'll find there has been incredibly supportive of me throughout my entire journey, and they will be there for you, too.

If you're *really* struggling, you might also consider seeing a professional counselor. I have. There's no shame in that. Having a licensed professional help you work through your fears and frustrations can do wonders for your overall well-being.

Above all else, give yourself a little grace. Remember, this is a marathon, not a sprint. You're in this for the long haul, and you're going to stumble every once in a while. We all do. And that's okay. It's part of the journey.

What you're going through isn't easy, but it is doable. Trust me, I've been there. In fact, I'm still there. And you know what? I'll always be here—right alongside you, cheering you on.

You can do this. Food saved me. And it can save you, too.

Acknowledgments

Special thanks to . . .

You, the reader: for being part of our community, which has grown and strengthened beyond what I ever expected over the last decade. Even though we may never meet each other in person, thank you for sharing your stories with me. Thank you for supporting my books and my work. Thank you for sharing them with your friends and loved ones with ailments, allergies, or autoimmune diseases. Thank you for being a part of my mission to change the world through food. Thank you for allowing me to be part of your families, in your kitchens and around your tables.

Ryan's and my parents: for stepping in whenever I am unable and Ryan is overstretched. It's been a long journey, and we couldn't be more thankful to have such loving grandparents for our children in such close proximity for the everyday, but especially for the times when we need our village.

Maria: for helping our children feel safe, loved, and in routine when I've been ill and incapacitated over the years.

Carol and the Tyndale editing team: for taking something from practically nothing and helping me turn it on its head so that it reflects my mission, speaks to my readers, and tells my story.

Kelli: for stepping in midway through the craziness to help streamline the process and ensure this book got to the finish line and out into the world.

Karen and Curtis: for your guidance and expertise as I fumbled my way through learning the "book-book" world and how drastically different it is from the cookbook world!

And finally, my deepest thanks to . . .

Ryan and the kids: for being my *why*. Thank you for being my reason to get out of bed every morning and my guiding light when I'm recovering from each flare-up. Thank you for sticking by me, caring for me, encouraging me, and loving me, even when I can't be all of myself. Because of you, I will never stop my quest for full healing. I pray that the day when I don't have to miss out on a single second of life comes very soon.

Grain-Free and Paleo Lists

What to Eat

- **FISH AND SHELLFISH** *(low-mercury and wild-caught; avoid farm-raised)*

- **MEATS** *(labeled 100% grass-fed when possible, or pasture-raised)*
    - beef
    - bison
    - lamb
    - pork

- **POULTRY** *(organic and pasture-raised)*
    - chicken
    - duck
    - turkey
    - eggs

- **BONE BROTH**

- **DARK, LEAFY GREENS**

- **FRUITS AND BERRIES**

- **FERMENTED FOODS**

- **HEALTHY OILS AND FATS**

- **NATURAL, UNREFINED SWEETENERS**

- **NUTS AND SEEDS**

- **SPICES AND DRIED HERBS**

- **VEGETABLES, EXCLUDING CORN AND WHITE POTATOES**

Key words to look for:

- 100 % grass-fed
- organic
- pasture-raised
- wild-caught
- natural
- local
- sustainable
- hormone-free
- antibiotic-free
- pesticide-free
- GMO-free

What to Avoid

- **GLUTEN**
  - barley
  - wheat
  - rye

- **GRAINS AND PSEUDOGRAINS**
  - amaranth
  - buckwheat
  - corn
  - durum
  - kamut
  - millet
  - oats
  - quinoa
  - rice
  - sorghum
  - spelt
  - teff
  - wheat (all varieties, including einkorn and semolina)
  - wild rice

- **LEGUMES**
  - beans
  - lentils
  - peanuts
  - soy

- **REFINED SUGAR, SUGAR SUBSTITUTES, AND SUGAR ALCOHOLS**

- **DAIRY**
  - cheese
  - cream
  - ice cream
  - milk
  - sour cream
  - whey
  - yogurt

- **ARTIFICIAL COLORINGS**

- **EMULSIFIERS**
  - carrageenan
  - cellulose gum
  - soy lecithin
  - xanthan gum

- **PROCESSED FOODS**

- **OTHER HIDDEN INGREDIENTS AND TERMS TO AVOID:**
  - agave nectar
  - cane sugar or juice
  - corn (syrup, high-fructose corn syrup, starch, dextrose, maltodextrin)
  - hydrogenated oils
  - modified food starch
  - monosodium glutamate (MSG)
  - seed oils such as canola, safflower, sunflower, soybean
  - sucrose, galactose, & maltose

Starting Grocery List

If you are transitioning to a gluten-free and grain-free diet, this grocery list includes the basics in each food group so you can stock your fridge and pantry.

- **PROTEIN** *(buy 100 percent grass-fed, organic, pasture-raised when possible)*
  - beef, bison, lamb, elk, etc.
  - poultry (turkey, chicken, duck, etc.)
  - pork
  - sausages, bacon, deli meat (without added sugars, carrageenan, nitrates, sulfates, and MSG)
  - fish and shellfish (wild-caught and fresh when possible)
  - eggs

- **VEGETABLES** *(organic, in season, and local when possible)*

  Including but not limited to:
  - acorn squash
  - artichoke
  - asparagus
  - beets
  - bell peppers
  - broccoli & broccoli rabe
  - brussels sprouts
  - butternut squash
  - cabbage
  - carrots
  - cauliflower
  - celery
  - cucumbers
  - eggplant
  - fennel
  - herbs
  - jicama
  - kabocha squash
  - kale
  - leeks
  - lettuce
  - mushrooms
  - parsley
  - parsnips
  - pumpkin
  - radishes
  - red onion
  - scallions
  - shallots
  - spaghetti squash
  - spinach
  - sweet potatoes
  - swiss chard
  - watercress
  - yam
  - yellow onion
  - zucchini

- **FRUITS** *(organic, in season, and local when possible)*
  - apples
  - apricots
  - avocados
  - bananas
  - berries
  - cantaloupe
  - cherries
  - dates
  - figs
  - grapefruit
  - grapes
  - lemons
  - limes
  - mangoes
  - nectarines
  - oranges
  - papaya
  - peaches
  - pears
  - pineapple
  - plums
  - pomegranates
  - raspberries
  - strawberries
  - tangerines
  - tomatoes
  - watermelon

- **FATS**
  - avocado oil
  - butter (grass-fed and pastured)
  - coconut oil (virgin or expeller-pressed for mild flavor)
  - duck fat
  - bacon fat
  - extra-virgin olive oil
  - ghee
  - lard (pastured)
  - macadamia oil
  - palm shortening (sustainable and organic)
  - sesame oil (toasted or cold pressed)
  - schmaltz
  - tallow

· BAKING INGREDIENTS

- almond flour (blanched)
- arrowroot flour
- baking powder (grain-free)
- baking soda
- cashew flour
- coconut crystals or palm sugar
- coconut flour
- cream of tartar
- pure dark maple syrup
- pure vanilla extract
- raw cacao powder or cocoa powder
- raw honey
- unsweetened or dark chocolate (at least 85% cacao; soy- and dairy-free)

· NUTS, SEEDS, AND NUT OR SEED BUTTERS
(purchase raw and organic when possible)

- almonds
- cashews
- flaxseeds
- hazelnuts
- macadamia nuts
- pecans
- pepitas (pumpkin seeds)
- pine nuts
- pistachios
- sesame seeds
- sunflower seeds
- walnuts
- almond butter
- cashew butter
- sunflower seed butter
- tahini

· LIQUIDS

- coconut milk (full-fat, canned)
- coconut water
- decaf coffee (Swiss water process)
- herbal tea
- nut milks: almond, cashew, pecan (free of carrageenan, gums, and sugar)
- organic coffee, in moderation

- **SEASONINGS**
  - fresh herbs
  - organic spices
  - sea salt or pink Himalayan salt

- **CONDIMENTS, JARRED AND CANNED GOODS**
  - avocado oil mayonnaise
  - ketchup (no sugar added or naturally sweetened)
  - mustards (no sugar added, preservative-free)
  - organic tomato products (no citric acid or sugars added)
    - diced tomatoes in juices
    - strained tomatoes or tomato puree
    - tomato paste
  - olives
  - curry paste
  - unsweetened applesauce
  - capers
  - pickles
  - fermented foods
    - sauerkraut
    - kimchi
    - water kefir
    - dairy-free yogurt
    - pickled vegetables
  - vinegars
    - apple cider
    - pure balsamic
    - champagne
    - red wine
  - fish sauce (Red Boat brand)
  - coconut aminos

· SNACKS
- · plantain chips
- · taro chips
- · grain-free tortilla chips
- · dried fruits (no sugar added or sweetened with fruit juices, and unsulfured)
- · seaweed (olive oil, sea salt)

Recipes

Chicken Stock (Bone Broth)

Prep time: 15 minutes · Cooking time: 18 hours · Yield: 8 to 10 cups

INGREDIENTS

4 pounds bone-in chicken parts and gizzards

10 to 12 cups filtered water

1 tablespoon apple cider vinegar

1 yellow onion, peeled and quartered

3 large carrots, cleaned and quartered

4 cloves garlic, smashed

2 stalks celery with leaves

2 bay leaves

1 teaspoon sea salt

½ teaspoon cracked black pepper

1 bunch fresh parsley

METHOD

1. Place chicken parts in a slow cooker and cover with just enough filtered water to barely immerse the bones. Cook on high for 2 hours.
2. Skim off any foam from the surface and remove the chicken. Shred the meat off the bones, and set the meat aside. Return the bones to the pot.
3. Reduce slow cooker to low. Add all the remaining ingredients, except the parsley, to the pot and cook on low for 16 hours or on high for 8 hours.
4. Turn off the pot, skim the fat off the top, stir in the parsley, and cover for 30 minutes.
5. Strain the broth through a fine-mesh sieve or cheesecloth. Store in the refrigerator for up to 2 weeks, or freeze for later use.

TIDBITS

- If you'd like the broth to have more flavor, cook the chicken ahead of time. Preheat oven to 450°F. Line a rimmed baking sheet with parchment paper and add the chicken. Drizzle chicken parts with 2 tablespoons avocado oil and sprinkle with 1 teaspoon sea salt. Roast the chicken for 30 to 40 minutes, until the skin is browned.
- If you are experiencing active digestive symptoms, try making this without the onions and garlic until symptoms are under control.

Chicken and Vegetable Soup

Prep time: 20 minutes · Cooking time: 12 minutes · Yield: 6 servings

INGREDIENTS

2 pounds bone-in, skin-on chicken breasts or thighs

6 cups Chicken Stock (Bone Broth) (see page 306)

1 yellow onion, chopped

3 cloves garlic, minced

3 teaspoons fine sea salt, plus more to taste

¾ teaspoon freshly ground black pepper, plus more to taste

6 celery stalks, sliced

6 carrots, sliced

1 small butternut squash, cubed

3 tablespoons chopped fresh flat-leaf parsley, or 1 tablespoon dried parsley

2 teaspoons dried turmeric powder

1½ tablespoons chopped fresh oregano, or 2½ teaspoons dried oregano

1½ teaspoons fresh thyme leaves, or ¾ teaspoon dried thyme

Zest of 1 lemon

1 teaspoon lemon juice

METHOD

1. Put the chicken in an electric pressure cooker. Add the bone broth, onion, garlic, salt, and pepper. Secure the lid, select the manual setting, and set it to high pressure for 20 minutes if using frozen chicken, or 10 minutes if using fresh chicken.

2. When the pressure cooker timer is done, quick release the pressure. Carefully take out the chicken. Remove the skin, shred the meat, and dispose of the bones. Return chicken to the pressure cooker.

3. Add the celery, carrots, butternut squash, parsley, turmeric, oregano, and thyme and season with salt and pepper to taste.

4. Secure the lid again, select the manual setting, and set it to high pressure for 2 minutes. Quick release the pressure.

5. Stir in the lemon zest and juice. Ladle soup into bowls and serve hot.

TIDBITS

- If you are experiencing active digestive symptoms, try making this without the onions and garlic until symptoms are under control.

- If using a slow cooker, add ingredients, then cover and cook on low for 6 hours.

Real-Deal Chocolate-Chip Cookies

Prep time: 12 minutes · Cooking time: 10 minutes · Yield: 1 dozen

INGREDIENTS

- ¼ cup sustainable palm shortening or grass-fed butter
- 1 egg at room temperature
- ¼ cup coconut sugar
- 2 tablespoons honey
- 2 teaspoons pure vanilla extract
- 1½ cups blanched almond flour
- 2 tablespoons coconut flour
- ½ teaspoon baking soda
- ½ teaspoon sea salt
- ¼ cup dark-chocolate pieces
- ¼ cup dairy-free chocolate chips

METHOD

1. Preheat the oven to 350°F.
2. Place the shortening and egg in a food processor and process for 15 seconds.
3. Add the coconut sugar, honey, and vanilla extract. Process again until combined.
4. Add the flours, baking soda, and salt, and process for 30 seconds.
5. Scrape down the sides and pulse again if necessary to fully incorporate the dry ingredients.
6. Stir in the chocolate by hand.
7. Use a large tablespoon to scoop balls of the dough, placing them on a baking sheet lined with parchment paper. Lightly press them down to flatten, making disks about ½-inch thick.
8. Bake for 10 minutes, until the cookies are browned around the edges. Cool on a wire rack.

Recipes on pages 308–312 first appeared in *Against All Grain: Delectable Paleo Recipes to Eat Well and Feel Great* (Las Vegas: Victory Belt Publishing, 2013). Used with permission of Victory Belt Publishing.

Blueberry Waffles

Prep time: 5 minutes · Cooking time: 15 minutes · Yield: 4 to 6 servings

INGREDIENTS

3 large eggs at room temperature

½ cup full-fat coconut milk

3 tablespoons honey or maple syrup

3 tablespoons coconut oil, melted

½ teaspoon pure vanilla extract

1 cup raw cashews or macadamia nuts

3 tablespoons coconut flour

¾ teaspoon baking soda

¼ teaspoon sea salt

½ cup blueberries

METHOD

1. Preheat a waffle iron to the lowest setting.
2. Place all the ingredients, except the blueberries, in a high-speed blender in the order listed.
3. Blend on low for 30 seconds, then increase to high and continue blending until the batter is completely smooth, about another 30 seconds.
4. Spoon the batter into the waffle iron, filling halfway and spreading evenly. Sprinkle a handful of blueberries over the batter.
5. Close the lid and cook for 45 seconds to 1 minute, until the steam stops rising from the machine and the waffle easily releases with a fork. Keep in a warm oven while you finish making the rest of the waffles.

TIDBITS

If you don't have a high-speed blender, grind the nuts in a food processor first. It may take a bit longer to blend, and you may have to use a spatula to scrape the batter down the sides of the jar to mix thoroughly.

Orange-Cranberry Muffins

Prep time: 10 minutes · Cooking time: 20–25 minutes · Yield: 12 muffins

INGREDIENTS

2 eggs at room temperature

¼ cup orange juice

2½ cups blanched almond flour

½ cup honey

½ cup sustainable palm shortening

1 tablespoon coconut flour

2 teaspoons pure vanilla extract

1 teaspoon orange zest

¾ teaspoon baking soda

½ teaspoon nutmeg

¼ teaspoon sea salt

1½ cups whole fresh cranberries

METHOD

1. Preheat the oven to 350°F.
2. Place a heatproof dish filled with 2 cups of water on the very bottom rack and position another rack in the center of the oven.
3. Place all the ingredients, except the cranberries, in a high-speed blender or food processor in the order listed and blend for 30 seconds. Scrape down the sides, then blend again until very smooth.
4. Stir in the cranberries by hand.
5. Grease a 12-cup muffin tin or line with paper cups. Spoon the batter into the cups, filling each ⅔ of the way full.
6. Place the muffins in the oven on the center rack and bake for 20 to 25 minutes, or until a toothpick inserted into the center of a muffin comes out clean.

TIDBITS

- These muffins can be assembled using only a blender or food processor—no mixing bowls!—so cleanup is fast.
- A steam bath (provided by the heatproof dish with water) helps the muffins rise and prevents the almond flour from browning while baking.

World-Famous Sandwich Bread

Prep time: 20 minutes · Cooking time: 50 minutes · Yield: 1 loaf

INGREDIENTS

Coconut oil for greasing pan

4 large eggs, separated

1 cup smooth, raw, unsweetened cashew butter

1 tablespoon honey

2½ teaspoons apple cider vinegar

¼ cup unsweetened almond milk

¼ cup coconut flour

1 teaspoon baking soda

½ teaspoon sea salt

METHOD

1. Preheat the oven to 300°F. Place a small heatproof dish of water on the bottom rack while the oven heats.
2. Line the bottom of an 8½-by-4½-inch loaf pan with parchment paper, then grease the sides of the pan with a very thin coating of coconut oil.
3. Place the egg whites in the bowl of a stand mixer and beat until soft peaks form, or use a hand mixer.
4. In a separate bowl, beat the egg yolks and cashew butter until combined, then mix in the honey, vinegar, and milk.
5. Sift the coconut flour, baking soda, and salt into the cashew butter mixture. Beat until combined.
6. Add 2 tablespoons of the whipped egg whites to the cashew butter mixture and beat until smooth. Add the remaining egg whites and beat on low until just combined. Do not overmix.
7. Pour the batter into the prepared loaf pan, then immediately put it into the oven.
8. Bake for 45 to 50 minutes, until the top is golden brown and a toothpick inserted into the center comes out clean.
9. Remove from the oven, then let cool for 15 to 20 minutes. Use a knife to free the sides from the loaf pan, then flip the pan upside down to release the loaf onto a cooling rack. Cool right side up for an hour before cutting.

TIDBITS

- The steam from the dish of water helps the loaf rise and keeps it a nice white color.

- While beating the eggs whites separately is not required, it helps the loaf rise to almost twice the size as adding the eggs whole.

- Use homemade cashew butter made from unsalted raw cashews or purchase raw, unsweetened cashew butter in a jar.

Endnotes

LOVE WELL

30 *"a persistent change in your bowel habits":* "Colon Cancer: Overview," Mayo Clinic, https://www.mayoclinic.org/diseases-conditions/colon -cancer/symptoms-causes/syc-20353669#:~:text=Signs%20and%20 symptoms%20of%20colon,as%20cramps%2C%20gas%20or%20pain.

30 *the number of young adults getting colon cancer:* Jessica B. O'Connell et al., "Rates of Colon and Rectal Cancers Are Increasing in Young Adults," *American Surgeon* 69, no.S 10 (October 2003): 866–72, https://pubmed .ncbi.nlm.nih.gov/14570365/.

38 *"involves inflammation and sores":* "Inflammatory Bowel Disease (IBD): Overview," Mayo Clinic, https://www.mayoclinic.org/diseases -conditions/inflammatory-bowel-disease/symptoms-causes/syc -20353315.

38 *Symptoms include "diarrhea":* "Inflammatory Bowel Disease (IBD)."

39 *One source I found said that well over one million people:* For a helpful fact book, see *The Facts about Inflammatory Bowel Diseases*, Crohn's and Colitis Foundation of America, November 2014, https://www.crohns colitisfoundation.org/sites/default/files/2019-02/Updated%20IBD %20Factbook.pdf.

39 *possible side effects of the medicines:* See "Prednisone Side Effects by Likelihood and Severity," WebMD, https://www.webmd.com/drugs /2/drug-6007-9383/prednisone-oral/prednisone-oral/details/list -sideeffects; "Prednisone," MedlinePlus, https://medlineplus.gov /druginfo/meds/a601102.html#side-effects.

40 *Sure enough: decreased awareness:* "Ambien Side Effects by Likelihood and Severity," WebMD, https://www.webmd.com/drugs/2/drug-9690 /ambien-oral/details/list-sideeffects.

58 *we don't need to "dread the disease":* Verse 6, NLT.

58 *"When pain surrounds":* Lyrics by Tim Hughes, "When Tears Fall," copyright © 2003, Thankyou Music/PRS.

71   *"you've experienced a molar pregnancy":* "Molar Pregnancy," Mayo Clinic, https://www.mayoclinic.org/diseases-conditions/molar-pregnancy/symptoms-causes/syc-20375175.

76–77   *Specific Carbohydrate Diet:* Elaine Gottschall, *Breaking the Vicious Cycle: Intestinal Health through Diet* (Baltimore: Kirkton Press, 1986).

EAT WELL

101   *nicotine patches, which studies had shown could suppress:* Vishmita Kannichamy et al., "Transdermal Nicotine as a Treatment Option for Ulcerative Colitis: A Review," *Cureus* 12, no. 10 (October 22, 2020): e11096, https://doi.org/10.7759/cureus.11096.

114   *"The Specific Carbohydrate Diet™ is predicated":* "Science behind the Diet," Breaking the Vicious Cycle," http://www.breakingthevicious cycle.info/p/science-behind-the-diet/.

115   *"The Specific Carbohydrate Diet™ is based on the principle":* "Science behind the Diet."

122   *It was harder than I expected:* One good outcome: This experience helped inspire my blog post "5 Tips to Save Money and Organize a Grain-Free Pantry," May 30, 2012, https://againstallgrain.com/2012/05/30/5-tips-to-save-and-organize-grain-free-pantry/.

LIVE WELL

192   *I did a bit of additional research on my own:* Brittany Buening, Sarah Hendrickson, and Christopher Smith, "Relationship between Pregnancy and Development of Autoimmune Diseases," *Journal of Women's Health, Issues and Care* 6, no. 1 (January 21, 2017), https:www.doi.org/10.4172/2325-9795.1000257; Vânia Vieira Borba et al., "Exacerbations of Autoimmune Diseases during Pregnancy and Postpartum," *Best Practice and Research Clinical Endocrinology and Metabolism* 33, no. 6 (December 2019), https://doi.org/10.1016/j.beem.2019.101321.

197   *"This is a hard post to write":* Excerpts from my blog post "Fighting a Flare," *Against All Grain*, May 21, 2016, https://againstallgrain.com/2016/05/21/fighting-ulcerative-colitis-flare-up/.

228–229   *"Today marks 3 weeks straight in bed":* Danielle Walker (@Danielle Walker), Instagram, February 28, 2018, https://www.instagram.com/p/BfwnRVMFTYS/?igshid=1r68ysgk2k83i.

249–250   *"I'm not going to sugarcoat it":* Danielle Walker (@Danielle Walker), Instagram, November 21, 2019, https://www.instagram.com/p/B5Il9HDBm9O/.

257   *people with chronic disease have a 75 percent divorce rate:* Alexandra Sifferlin, "Divorce More Likely When Wife Falls Ill," *Time*, May 1, 2014, https://time.com/83486/divorce-is-more-likely-if-the-wife-not-the-husband-gets-sick/#:~:text=Some%20numbers%20show%20the%20that,chronic%20disease%20end%20in%20divorce.&text=The%20researchers%20also%20looked%20for,than%20women%20to%20get%20sick.

About the Author

DANIELLE WALKER is a *New York Times* bestselling cookbook author (*Against All Grain*, *Meals Made Simple*, *Celebrations*, and *Eat What You Love*), health advocate, and self-trained chef. After being diagnosed with an autoimmune disease at age twenty-two and suffering for many years, Danielle found health through dietary and lifestyle changes. Inspired by what she has learned on her own health journey, Danielle shares her gluten-free recipes on her blog at daniellewalker.com as a beacon of hope for others.

For over a decade she has been a pioneer in advocating for a grain- and gluten-free lifestyle, having earned a spot on the coveted Forbes 30 under 30 list in 2015. Her delicious recipes have satiated the palates of autoimmune sufferers, kids with food allergies, healthy eaters, and foodies alike. From nostalgic comfort foods to healthy holiday swaps to quick-and-easy meals for kids, Danielle has created thousands of recipes as well as kitchen, food, and parenting hacks that make life easier and healthier.

Danielle regularly shares her health journey, recipes, and expert tips on the *Today* show, *The Doctors*, *E! News*, *Access Hollywood*, *Home & Family*, and many other nationally syndicated shows. Her work has been featured in *People*, *O Magazine*, *USA Today*, *Shape*, *Women's Health*, *Parents*, *Well + Good*, and more.

More by Danielle Walker

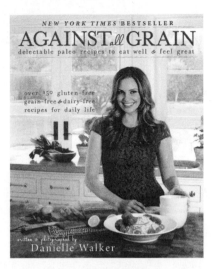

Against All Grain:
Delectable Paleo Recipes
to Eat Well & Feel Great

VICTORY BELT PUBLISHING

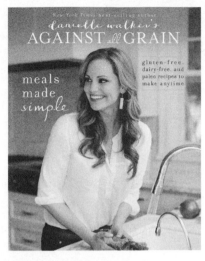

Danielle Walker's Against All Grain:
Meals Made Simple: Gluten-Free, Dairy-Free,
and Paleo Recipes to Make Anytime

VICTORY BELT PUBLISHING

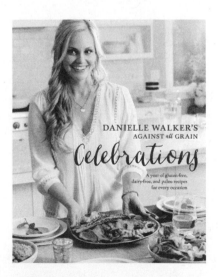

Danielle Walker's Against All Grain
Celebrations: A Year of Gluten-Free,
Dairy-Free, and Paleo Recipes
for Every Occasion

TEN SPEED PRESS

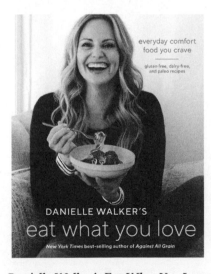

Danielle Walker's Eat What You Love:
Everyday Comfort Food You Crave;
Gluten-Free, Dairy-Free,
and Paleo Recipes

TEN SPEED PRESS

Food saved me from the stress of endless medical appointments and the myriad of medications that halted any long term-healing.—Sabrina Food saved me from feeling isolated due to food sensitivities.—Briana G Food saved me from suffering with stage 4 endometriosis!—Jess T Food saved me from thyroid cancer, Lyme disease, and celiac.—Carly C Food saved me from Crohn's disease. It saved me from further gut damage. My own food choices have saved my family as well, and I would like to believe that it has added many more (healthy) years to our lives.—Maryana S Food saved me by being a vehicle to show my love for my tribe.—Lauren B Food saved me from debilitating stomach pain.—Cassia N Food saved me from chronic fatigue syndrome and debilitating inflammation. Food saved me from having to live a gray life. I learned how to cook colorfully and even enjoy my favorite chocolate chip cookies!—Abby C Food saved me by changing my life to be a better wife and mother.—Ashley M Food saved me by putting my Crohn's in remission. By dropping all inflammatory markers within months. Now, with a son diagnosed with juvenile arthritis, I knew where to turn to do our part in his healing.—Heather K Food saved me when I went from being a fit and active 38-year-old woman to a woman who felt like she had the body of a 90-year-old in less than two months of my

Food saved me from having to be on medication
for the rest of my life. It also helped me conceive;
I now have an amazing daughter who brings
me so much joy every day!–Monique B

diagnosis with rheumatoid arthritis. I couldn't move in the mornings and at one point couldn't dress myself. Then I found an autoimmune Paleo diet, and after 90 days my inflammation was 80 percent gone. I got my life back, and though things weren't so dramatically different from the life I had before my diagnosis, food gave me hope. I also adopted a new way of living, focusing on supplements, working on stress and relationships, and exercising! But food started my healing journey, and I'm grateful for it.—Ginger H Food saved me from having to be on medication for the rest of my life. It also helped me conceive; I now have an amazing daughter who brings me so much joy every day!—Monique B Food saved me from my Crohn's disease.—Brynnen L Food saved me by helping my (seemingly) never-ending flare-up from Crohn's, pyoderma gangrenosum, and hidradenitis suppurativa to finally end. I can live my life again. After almost two years of being sick and in pain nonstop, my lifestyle changes in my diet helped nurse me back to life. I'll never take anything for granted again.—Kristen H Food saved me from celiac disease and autoimmune dermatological reactions.—Sarah H Food saved me because we learned that going gluten-free and dairy-free could help our autistic child. . . . Through the journey of food, we now have a fully verbal, typical, beautiful, thriving teenage son.—Lisa W

Food saved me from hormonal imbalances that were destroying my mood, self-esteem, and general health. Food saved me from a heavy weight of sadness too (because food is a big part of my memories and because cooking is FUN).—Karlie M Food saved me from Crohn's disease. Food saved me from giving up so I can be there for my daughter.—Corey J Food saved me and my daughter Megan from Hashimoto's. I have all of Danielle's cookbooks (one of them signed!). Danielle helped us get back to living life and enjoying it again!—Christine P Food saved me three years ago when my world changed after a gangrenous gallbladder almost killed me. It damaged so much of my insides, and everything I ate made me sick. I had been following Danielle for a while but never really paid attention to the reasons behind the recipes until I was in a position where I would try anything to get my life back. The recipes and advice on going through not only my illness but also everyday life are what helped save my life!—Leslie M Food saved me from chronic autoimmune issues including lifelong hypothyroidism, allergies, and asthma.—Marci P Food saved me by managing my idiopathic anaphylactic reactions. My body used to trigger an anaphylactic reaction for no known reason a few times a month. The doctors said it was just something my body did, but a functional medicine provider taught me how to reduce the

Food saved me from debilitating migraines
and from missing out on precious moments
with my kids and husband.–Charlsie G

inflammation in my body through diet. After being gluten/dairy-free for seven and a half years, I now have a reaction only about once a year.—Diane H Food saved me from continued pain every single month after being diagnosed at 34 with endometriosis.—Julie D Food saved me from losing my connection with friends and family.—Melissa V Food saved me from migraines. Danielle has been my lifeline for so long. I even gave her cookbook to my student's parents when they discovered she had major food allergies!—Kate C Food saved me from mysterious lymphatic inflammation (and from an invasive biopsy) just in time for my wedding.—Carol S Food saved me from giving up and giving in to the symptoms of chronic illness.—Jacklyn G Food saved me from my crippling and overwhelmingly sudden anxiety. Desperate for a solution, I stumbled across research about how eating a gluten- and dairy-free diet can help reset your gut, which I firmly believe is deeply connected to mental health. Danielle taught me that with a few simple swaps, you can still eat and make delicious, healthy food. Food is medicine! I am proud to say that I never had to use anxiety medication because I decided to try this natural solution first. And it worked.—Paulina V Food saved me from MS. Food saved me by giving me the confidence to get in the kitchen where I learned how to cook while knowing it's OK to mess up recipes!—Jennifer G